Keep
Your Heart
Running

Keep Your Heart Running

A graduated,
total health and
fitness program
for people of
all ages

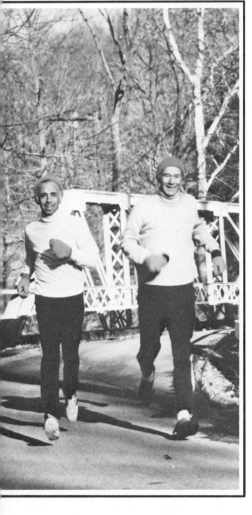

Paul J. Kiell, M.D. and
Joseph S. Frelinghuysen

Winchester Press

Library of Congress Cataloging in Publication Data

Kiell, Paul J
    Keep your heart running.

    Bibliography: p.
    Includes index.
    1. Exercise. 2. Physical fitness. 3. Hygiene.
I. Frelinghuysen, Joseph Sherman, 1912–   joint
author. II. Title. [DNLM: 1. Gymnastics.
2. Physical fitness—Popular works. QT255 K48k]
RA781.K52   613.7   76-27249
ISBN 0-87691-182-3

Published by Winchester Press
205 East 42nd Street, New York, N.Y. 10017

Printed in the United States of America

WINCHESTER is a Trademark of Olin Corporation used by Winchester Press,
Inc., under authority and control of the Trademark Proprietor

Chapter 1

Page 5 (captions), from *Scientific Principles and Methods of Strength Fitness,*
by John Patrick O'Shea. Copyright © 1969 by Addison-Wesley Publishing
Company, Inc., Reading, Mass. Used by permission of Addison-Wesley
Publishing Company.

Page 5 (pictures), from *Atlas of Men,* by Dr. William H. Sheldon. Copyright ©
1954 by Harper & Row. Used by arrangement with William Sheldon, 1970,
Hafner Publishing Company, Inc., Darien, Conn.

Chapter 3

Page 24, from *The Collected Works of C. G. Jung,* edited by G. Adler,
M. Fordham, H. Read, and W. McGuire, translated by R. F. C. Hull. Bollingen

Series XX, Vol. 6, *Psychological Types,* copyright © 1971 by Princeton University Press. Used by permission of Princeton University Press.

Chapter 4

Page 31, from *Road Racers and Their Training,* edited by Joe Henderson. Used by permission of Tafnews Press, Los Altos, Calif., 1970.

Page 31, from *Your Heart and How to Live With It,* by Dr. Lawrence E. Lamb. Copyright © 1969 by Lawrence E. Lamb. Used by permission of the Viking Press, Inc.

Chapter 5

Page 33, from *The Physiological Effects of Exercise Programs on Adults,* 1968, by Thomas K. Cureton. Used by permission of Charles C. Thomas and Dr. Thomas K. Cureton.

Chapter 6

Pages 60–63, from *Miss Craig's 21-Day Shape-Up Program for Men and Women,* by Marjorie Craig. Copyright © 1968 by Random House, Inc. Used by permission of Random House, Inc.

Chapter 7

Pages 79, 80, and 104 reprinted from *Bur Courses for Adjustable Weights,* the Bur Barbell Co., Inc. (uncopyrighted publication).

Chapter 8

Page 128 (picture), from *Vigor for Men over 30,* by Warren R. Guild, Stuart D. Cowan, Samm Sinclair Baker. Copyright © 1967 by the Macmillan Company. Used by permission of the Macmillan Company.

Chapter 9

Page 158, from *Medical Tribune,* New York, New York, October 24, 1970. Copyright © Medical Tribune, Inc. Used by permission of Medical Tribune, Inc.

Chapter 11

Page 194, from *The Treatment of Renal Failure,* by John P. Merrill, M.D. Copyright © 1965 by Grune & Stratton, Inc., New York, N. Y. Used by permission of Dr. John P. Merrill.

Page 198, from *The Complete Walker,* by Colin Fletcher. Copyright © by Colin Fletcher. Used by permission of Alfred A. Knopf, Inc.

Chapter 12

Page 218, from *The Hurricane Years,* by Cameron Hawley. Copyright © 1968 by Cameron Hawley. Used by permission of Little, Brown and Company.

Contents

Acknowledgments

Our sincere thanks go to the Harvard School of Public Health, especially to the Guggenheim Center for Aerospace Health and Safety and the Department of Nutrition; and individually to Dr. Ross A. McFarland, Guggenheim Professor Emeritus of Aerospace Health and Safety. Long on patience and understanding of his fellow humans, Dr. McFarland has been the good friend and mentor of this work. In addition, our particular gratitude goes to Emily F. McFarland for her comprehensive and highly competent editorial review of the manuscript.

Our deep appreciation is extended to Dr. William V. Beshlian for his perceptive and invaluable comments on the manuscript, which expressed the human as well as the medical aspects of his clinical experience.

We express our thanks to Dr. Frederick J. Stare, Dr. Jean Mayer, and Dr. J. Mark Hegsted, for their help in answering many questions. Also, our thanks go to Dr. Howard W. Stoudt, for his guidance in anthropometry and to Mr. John C. Loring, librarian, and Miss Toula Coules for their assistance.

We are pleased to acknowledge our indebtedness to Dr. Kenneth H. Cooper for having drawn heavily on his splendid work in the field of "Aerobics." Dr. Cooper, formerly colonel, USAF-MC, now runs The Cooper Clinic, The Aerobics Activity Center, and the Institute for Aerobics Research in Dallas, which are devoted to the most advanced procedures in preventive medicine.

For many papers and replies to correspondence, as well as for reviewing Chapter 11 on fluid and electrolyte management, we are grateful to Dr. Richard L. Westerman, Senior Clinical Research Physician, Upjohn International, Inc., and Dr. Gerard Balakian, Department of Internal Medicine and Chairman of the Pharmacy Committee, Englewood Hospital, Englewood, N.J. and Coordinator in the Adverse Drug Reaction Program of the F.D.A.

We express our appreciation to Dr. Warren R. Guild for his encouragement in both the physical training and literary fields, and also special thanks go to Margaret Michel and Elizabeth Mihaly. Their painstaking editing, checking of references, and typing have saved us many hours and have produced a far more readable and intelligible text.

Authors'
Note

Although there is considerable scientific and medical material behind this book, it has been written in layman's language wherever possible in hope that the everyday expression will have more appeal to the nonscientific reader. However, a few interesting, but somewhat technical words have been included, so a brief glossary has been added.

To avoid overburdening the text, references, interviews and letters are listed by chapter at the end of the book. Statements not directly supported by the references are simply the authors' opinions based on experience and observation.

Foreword

During twenty-five years in the practice of internal medicine and clinical cardiology, I have become increasingly interested in exercise as a means of promoting general health, and have encouraged it for patients with no limiting or debilitating medical problems.

With this in mind, I have reviewed many exercise books, most of which have had a limited approach, recommending either calisthenics, weight training, or some form of aerobic exercise. These books usually say, "Do twenty of this, ten of that," or another will say, "Jog so far and increase it every week." From the point of view of the overall health and well-being of the whole person, each of these tells only a minor part of the entire diet, weight control and exercise story. This means the patient would have to read three or four books to get a complete program.

Keep Your Heart Running appealed to me in the way it deals with the whole nutritional, physical, and mental environment and because each of the authors brings to this book his own special brand of credentials. One, a physician in his mid-forties, who specializes in psychiatry, prescribes his own therapy with daily eight to ten mile runs during his lunch period. The other, after thirty-five years of sedentary living, went on this program for two years and then completed the Boston Marathon at the age of fifty-seven. While I have no intention of telling my patients to read this book and go out and run twenty-six miles, I do feel that this man's own experience was the test of the validity of the program. At the present time the authors have finished twenty marathons between them in the past few years and are happily and irrevocably hooked on their program.

Keep Your Heart Running's broad approach to health has great value for the average layman. In an uncomplicated way the authors explain why people should exercise, giving them some simple physiology to help their understanding of the subject. The chapter on physical activity includes exercises to build up and maintain adequate strength for the daily tasks plus others to develop flexibility. These are combined with sensible aerobic exercise to increase the ability of the heart to tolerate stress. This is of special concern to me as a medical doctor.

Many of the freak diets that have been published in recent years are nonsense. Some are even dangerous. Therefore, these authors' diet was like a breath of fresh air. Their study of the medical and scientific literature on nutrition has been thorough. Their conclusions from it are accurate and they present a sound and well-expressed nutritional program. If the person with no medical restrictions will use this diet, both his physical health and mental outlook should benefit from it.

The subject of fluid and electrolyte balance has received too little attention. Even today, I know a few athletic coaches who could read this book to advantage, because they still adhere to that absurdity about not permitting athletes to take fluids during strenuous exercise. However, well-informed professional athletes are now using electrolyte fluids routinely during active participation. This chapter should be a help and safeguard for the warm-weather and long-duration exercisers.

To those individuals without any of the medical limitations I have referred to above, I can recommend this book without hesitation. It has built-in safeguards to avoid the inherent dangers of change from a sedentary to an active life. It explains about checking the heart rate and about losing weight gradually and not on a crash basis. I particularly like the idea that the program should be done for fun and not taken as a dose of medicine and emphatically agree that it should be for life and not an off and on affair.

WILLIAM V. BESHLIAN, M.D.

Introduction

If you were suddenly asked, "Is your health as important to you as your automobile?" wouldn't you think the speaker had taken leave of his senses? Nevertheless, many of us spend more time and money to keep our cars going than we spend on our health.

Car expenses are inevitable, but medical bills can sometimes be avoided or at least minimized by a simple, inexpensive program that takes only minutes, not hours a day. In addition, it will give you the best possible chances of escaping both the doctor's bills and the grief that goes with them. Remember, too, that you can get spare parts for your car, but the parts replacement problem for your body is years from a solution.

If you want to find out about your health right now, try this little test and see how you've been taking care of it.

Assuming you haven't just raced your twelve-year old son around the block, lie down and rest for a few minutes; then take your pulse at one of these two points: Grasp your wrist from the back so your middle finger comes just over the big bone on the thumb side, about an inch or so away from the joint, or gently press your index finger close in front of your ear just below the side part of the cheekbone. Feel the pulse beat? Now place your watch so you can see the second hand and count the beat for 15 seconds and multiply by 4. Stand up and count it again. If the answer is 50 lying down and 60 standing up for a man, and 55 and 65 for a woman, it is either low because something is wrong or because you are in marvelous shape—and you should find out from the doctor which it is.

On the other hand, a rate in the upper 70s or 80s, lying down, is never good because your pulse rate is the indicator of how hard your heart has to work when it's idling just enough to get its normal housekeeping done (basal metabolism). Usually if the beat is high, you have the equivalent of rust in your pipes, bad equipment somewhere, or you've been stoking up with too much alcohol, tobacco, coffee, tea, or a poor diet. For this, too, you should visit your doctor to find out the causes.

Most people who have been on this type of program for a number of years have pulse rates of 45–50 lying down and 55–60 standing. (Pulse rates usually go up a little in the evening.) Some champion athletes have resting pulse rates in the 30s. So, barring any illness, a low rate is a sign of fitness and good health, and the reduction of yours is one of the objectives of this book. Other objectives of equal importance are to increase your enjoyment of living, to enhance your natural abilities, and to help you make better use of your knowledge and training in your chosen vocation.

Somewhere in our genetic endowment there is a natural resistance to physical activity, which, because of necessity, remained buried for thousands of years. But only recently it has bounded to the surface to have a Roman holiday with those symbols of affluence that have become instigators of physical inactivity. This book attempts to overcome the resistance to physical activity, wherever it lies, by offering rewards that are so great they have to be experienced to be believed. This is part of the difficulty. The first steps have to be taken on faith, plus plenty of suggestion and enticement.

There is an increasing number of athlete doctors who occasionally ridicule the pre-exercise medical exam, saying exercise is not dangerous because it is a natural thing and we were meant to do it. The career that is really dangerous, they say, is a sedentary life, so if you are going to embark on one, you must first have a medical exam.

Even though there is some truth to their tongue-in-cheek remark, we still recommend very strongly taking a medical exam before embarking on an exercise program. It is a screening for trouble caused by past neglect that is as yet undetected. So visit your personal physician and tell him your plans and ask him to give you a complete medical examination to find out if he will approve. (If the doctor you see is not your regular physician, he will surely ask your medical history and that of your family, which is particularly important with regard to presence of heart disease.)

Principal features of the examination are resting pulse rate, blood pressure, blood serum analysis, breathing (vital capacity) and a resting electrocardiogram to detect any obvious or subclinical signs of coronary heart disease. Any complicating factors, such as high blood pressure, high cholesterol, or triglycerides, should be identified and medical and nutritional remedies prescribed. Steps to eliminate manifest problems, such as cigarette smoking and overweight, could be undertaken as part of the program in this book.

Assuming you have passed the above tests, it is most important for you to take a treadmill stress test to detect any occult or asymptomatic heart disease. (For an up-to-date list of Stress Testing Facilities, write to: The National Jogging Association, 1910 K St. N.W., Suite 202, Washington, D.C. 20006, Attention: B.S. Woods.) Everyone has heard about the man who just had his annual checkup, was given a clean bill of health and suddenly died or became seriously ill from a heart attack. The objective of this treadmill stress test, which can now be monitored and interpreted by new and highly sophisticated methods, is to detect the occult coronary or similar disease that undoubtedly causes the unfortunate type of incident mentioned above.

If you are in sufficiently good health to be approved, some doctors will grant it with more enthusiasm than others. With the amount of published statistical evidence today, indicating the benefits of such a program, it would indeed be discouraging to hear: "What are you trying to prove?" or, "Why don't you just relax and take it easy?" If you have passed your physical and this is the answer, these authors must strongly disagree. Twenty, or even ten years ago this was the classic advice to the overworked, overweight, oversmoked, and overnervous business person. It is hoped that this will not be the case today, especially when the Committee on Exercise of the American

Heart Association believes that "regular, vigorous exercise enhances the quality of life by increasing the physical capability for work and play."

Assuming, however, that you have seen your doctor and received an affirmative response, the first two or three weeks of the program may be difficult. The best way to start is to consider only one day's activity at a time. Then, as you begin that, think only of the immediate step you are about to take. Next, remember the thing you do best in life and say to yourself, "If I'm so good at that, I'm sure I can do this program, which is difficult, but probably easier than my own thing at which I am an expert."

Good luck! Put your faith and trust in the program, particularly during those first few challenging weeks. After that it will become much easier and you'll start to enjoy it.

P.J.K.
J.S.F.

Keep
Your Heart
Running

1 | The Shape

Have you ever seen a moving picture of yourself in a bathing suit? Outside of the Hollywood and TV crowd, most of whom have pretty good figures, not too many of us have. It's far more revealing than a snapshot and a dreadful shock if it doesn't coincide with your image of yourself.

At home movies you've heard violent protests, "That can't be me! I don't look like that!"

But yes you do—the movie camera tells the truth and frequently it's very upsetting. A good self-image and the knowledge that others have a good image of us are deeply important and are basic to a sense of pride and well-being. If this turns out to be another of life's illusions, we must convert the damage to our pride into an incentive and motivating drive toward getting a good image honestly restored.

First, you should try to find the answer to the question, "Really and truly, how do I look to others?" Take off all your clothes and, with a hand mirror, look at yourself sideways in a full-length mirror. You may get such a nasty jolt that you can't believe it's you, since this indirect view is somehow much more revealing than staring at yourself directly. When you have recovered, think of your favorite athlete, possibly a champion swimmer or runner. You will probably be able to decide pretty quickly whether or not you come even close to their lean and shapely figures.

Next, try to imagine how much you would have to lose to be as slim and trim as they are. Even so, loss of weight alone may not do it, because these people work hard on tough programs to look the way they do. If you don't have a shape like one of your idols, whether by inheritance or from the way you eat and live, this book's objective is to help you acquire it as expeditiously as possible. With that in view, we should first have a look at some of the characteristics with which nature has endowed you.

There are three basic types of figures, with an infinite variety of gradations and combinations between them. Basically, these types are endomorph, mesomorph, and ectomorph, as shown on page 5. If you recognize yourself clearly as one type or another, no amount of effort on your part is going to change that type any more than you can change the color of your eyes. Although it is more difficult for an endomorph to look like an athlete, less so for a mesomorph, and easy for an ectomorph, you can present what you have in its best possible light. With the satisfaction of knowing that you have done the best possible for your natural endowment, you will have solved one of the riddles

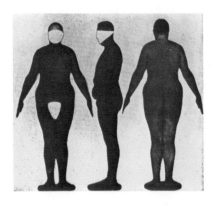

Endomorph: Soft muscu-
lature, round face, short
neck, double chin, and
wide hips. Heavy fat pads,
distributed on back of the
upper arms, hips, abdomen,
buttocks, and thighs.
Trunk, arms, and breast
tend to be somewhat
feminine.

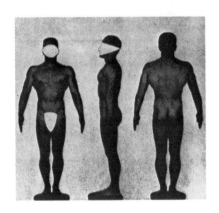

Mesomorph: Solid, mus-
cular, big-boned physique,
characterized by square-
ness, hardness, and rugged-
ness. Mesomorphs are
generally medium in height,
possess large chests, slender
waists, long torsos, rela-
tively short, powerful legs
and arms.

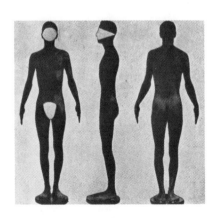

Ectomorph: Slender body,
short trunk, and long legs
and arms. Ectomorphs also
tend to have long, narrow
feet and hands, long slender
necks, narrow chests, and
very little fat.

of identity and the self-image problem. It doesn't take a million dollars and a lot of brass. With just a fine figure, good posture, and a few nice clothes fitted to your new shape, this new identity of yours will blossom like a rose.

2 | Our Way of Life

"No machines will increase the
possibilities of life. They only
increase the possibilities
of idleness."

John Ruskin: *Fors Clavigera,*
Letter V

If you were not happy about your appearance in the mirror, it is important to realize how machines of all kinds have changed our lives and figures by greatly reducing our activity. Machine technology is advancing at an increasingly rapid rate and threatens to engulf us unless we learn to live with it both physically and emotionally. But learning to live with it does not mean being enslaved by it so that it becomes an objective in itself that sets our standards of value based on this special brand of materialism.

Our suggestions throughout this book for keeping healthy and happy in our unfulfilling mechanical environment are new in the context of the recent groundswell of interest in outdoor and physical activity, but in another sense they are very old, older even than Juvenal's "Our prayers should be for a sound mind in a healthy body." To achieve this adjustment we don't advocate fighting the technology, which would be turning the clock back, but instead, fighting the all-pervasive inactivity that is its inevitable by-product.

Our resistance to activity has teamed up with the technology so that doing things the easy way has become a way of life. Many of the ads seen in the media are oriented toward labor-saving, step-saving devices, and even short cuts to wealth. These are supposed to save time and energy. For what? In order to dash from one meaningless activity to another? To jump in a car and go on trivial errands, get on a riding lawn mower to mow one-tenth of an acre of grass, or tear around on the snow on caterpillar-driven sleds? Eventually, life becomes a frenetic series of methods, where the method becomes the end and the objective in itself, rather than the accomplishment of something worthwhile.

These technological "advances" have reduced our daily physical output so that many people burn less food than they eat, creating a surplus that gets stored as fat. The following list shows for each gadget the calories that would be burned if the work were done by hand or on foot. These represent our daily calorie surplus.

This mixture of labor-saving devices, machinery, and gadgets is part "his" and part "hers." Since most of us use a lot of these things, an average estimate of at least one-fourth of the total calorie surplus (109 calories per day) probably applies to you. Multiplying by 365 days gives 39,785 calories per year. At approximately 3,600 calories to the pound, this is equal to 11 pounds, which you can put on in a year. Unless you step up your physical activity in some

THE CALORIE SURPLUS CREATED
BY TECHNOLOGY
(As compared to 50 years ago)

*Daily Calorie Surplus**

In the House

Live in ranch house instead of 2–3 story house	20
(10 trips upstairs a day at 2 calories)	
Extra telephone extension (5 calls a day)	5
TV set—reduction in activity	25
TV set with remote control switch—extra reduction	3
in activity	
Electric dishwasher	40
Electric clothes washer	40
Electric clothes dryer	18
Kitchen—Electric mixer	5
Electric blender	5
Electric carving knife	2
Vacuum cleaner—one-half hour, twice a week	35
Premixed and processed foods, instead of homemade	20
Store bread, instead of homebaked, twice a week	30
Electric toothbrush	1
Electric carpentry tools—drill, sander, etc.	4
Electric shoe polisher	10
Overheated house in winter	10

The Car

Electric windows	2
Power steering	10
Power brakes	5

* Where applicable, energy values were adapted from references listed for the Appendix. Others, which were estimated, may be subject to some modification, but on the average they are probably not too far off. The purpose of this table, however, is to show the reduction in activity caused by mechanization, with its inevitable effects on our figures and fatness.

Used for short errands, mail, forgotten groceries, etc.   20
Take it to car wash, instead of doing it yourself   5

Outside the House

Power mower in summer; power shovel and plow in   30
    winter
Power clippers and trimmers   5
Power saw (infrequent use)   .   2

To and From Work, At Work, Shopping

Buses or taxis for short hauls   20
Escalator   5
Elevator   10
Electric adding machine   2
Electric typewriter   6
Electric pencil sharpener   1

Recreation Time

Winter—Using skidoo or ski lift—5 weekends averaged   20
    over the year (instead of walking or climbing)
Summer—Using golf cart or motor bike   20
                                                      Total: 436

way to offset it, in four to five years you will be grossly and dangerously overweight.

In this concept of life style in relation to the human heart and blood vessels, Dr. Michael DeBakey has said: "Man was made to work, and work hard, I don't think it ever hurt anyone." This seems clearly to mean both mental and physical work, and also that the cardiovascular system expects to be worked hard and is better off for it. But besides Dr. DeBakey, why do Drs. Kenneth H. Cooper, Herman K. Hellerstein, John L. Boyer, Per-Olof Åstrand,

Bengt Saltin, and many other distinguished people in the medical and scientific field say this? In order to try to answer this question, let's first look back at what has gone into our human makeup.

"Know then thyself, presume not God to scan;
The proper study of mankind is man."

Alexander Pope:
An Essay on Man, II.i.

For a long time after Darwin thrust his shocking theories on an unsuspecting world, many scientists liked to pretend that we have descended from a peace-loving simian who wouldn't hurt a fly. Then one day Raymond Dart, a Johannesburg anatomy professor, discovered a hominid, which he named *Australopithecus Africanus.* His discovery was later expanded by Louis and Mary Leakey and their son Richard, East African anthropologists, who upset the peace-loving applecart. Their nasty little hominid, who was found in the Olduvai Gorge in Tanzania, only weighed 80 to 100 pounds, but the evidence has indicated he was, variously, carnivorous, herbivorous, and highly predatory, even against his own species.

In some way this creature's ancestors had survived the terrible droughts and swirling dust storms of the Pliocene for millions of years. The australopithecine who emerged in Central and South Africa was a hardy runner, who outwitted and outfought in packs fierce predators, and ran down and slaughtered for food the lesser creatures that roamed the plains.

The Victorians had a hard time with these apelike ancestors who were foisted on them by Darwin. One lady said that she hoped it wasn't true; but if it was, she prayed it wouldn't become generally known. Others fervently hoped they would go away. But the fact is they haven't. With each new discovery they appear more surely in the direct line of human ancestry, and whether we like it or not, we have come from the toughest, most resourceful, and certainly the most predatory, mammalians that have ever stalked the face of the earth.

A strange reminder of the incredible endurance of these ancient creatures survives today in the Barranca del Cobre of the remote Sierra Madre Occidental of Mexico. It is the Tarahumara Indians, a peaceful Uto-Aztec tribe, whose men and women can run enormous distances over very difficult terrain. They run as a sport in races, in which they kick a wooden ball for distances over a hundred miles for a period of two or three days. For a livelihood, they run after deer and wild turkeys, which finally drop from exhaustion and are killed.

Despite pains in their legs and abdominal cramps from dehydration, the Tarahumara Indians are so overcome with the enthusiasm of the race or hunt that they rarely feel the pain. Afterwards they do have complaints, but are compensated by having achieved a special popularity with the women. One wonders to what extent the competitors are able to relish this popularity after running a hundred miles.

Where did these fascinating people come from? Is it possible that they somehow escaped the spreading Sahara and Arabian deserts of the Pliocene and crossed the Atlantic Ocean on crude rafts, driven from Africa by a terrible famine? Anthropologists tell us that as the lush greenery of the Miocene savannah and forests vanished, all living things suffered horribly. During the ensuing Pliocene, twelve million years of drought changed the face of the

African continent and every creature had to change its way of life or perish.

One way or the other, we ourselves are descended from people who had extraordinary stamina and endurance, and we have inherited cardiovascular and endocrine systems which react in the same way as theirs. Prolonged, stressful physical activity was as much a part of the lives of our ancestors as eating and sleeping, and today it is still as necessary as the other two needs.

The conditioning of our habits over the last seventy-five years by technological "advances," which have all but eliminated physical activity, is totally at odds with our ancestry. We take so many things for granted that we live an existence for which our bodies, created to withstand heavy and often violent physical output, are not suited. Without compensatory activity, we end up by being overweight, ill, miserable, or all three.

Early man's responses to emotions such as fear, rage, and pain were put there to help him meet challenges. Usually, these were met by violent attack or flight, which used up the adrenalines produced by the response, but in Western society, it isn't acceptable to respond by violence or escape. If someone threatens us, we must keep our cool, so that the basic response, which was intended to be protective, is aborted by lack of physical activity. Therefore, we sit and seethe, causing more adrenal energy, which eventually harms us both physically and mentally.

One never learns anything much from ease and comfort. Their by-product is malaise, a dissatisfaction that stems from a sense of nonfulfillment, which is a forerunner of mood depression. The great teachers are hardship, duress, and suffering—from these we can learn a great deal about ourselves as well as other people. The man or

woman who has experienced a misfortune can com-
municate understanding. The one who hasn't feels uncomfortable in the face of his friends' troubles because he does
not know how to convey sympathy and understanding. In
the physical analogy, stress increases the body's ability to
adapt to hardship through increased strength and endurance.

The degree of inactivity to which Americans have become accustomed was most apparent to one of the authors
when, in the Second World War, after escaping from a
prison camp, he stayed with European mountain families
whose houses had no light, heat, water, or plumbing. They
had a roof, four heavy stone walls, and a huge fireplace.
For them, the meaning of life was the business of existence; up some days at four o'clock to bake bread and on
their feet working steadily until nine at night. The man
ploughed his mountainside patch of ground with a bullock,
planted by hand, and with the help of his family harvested
by hand. They ground the grain themselves or took it a long
distance to the mill and back. The rewards were a meager
existence, eked out year after year. Always tired, and
nearly always hungry, they managed somehow to handle
degrees of disappointment and frustration that would cause
many American families to disintegrate.

Certainly no one advocates a return to a primitive existence, because we have obviously achieved better education, medical expertise, and worldwide communications.
We don't die of measles and chicken pox any more, but we
have become prey to a host of inactivity diseases. Dr. Jean
Mayer, distinguished Professor of Nutrition at Harvard
from 1950 to 1976, is a Frenchman by birth. He has stated
that by coming to America to live he has, at least statisti-

cally, increased his chances of having a heart attack by 400 percent. His reasoning is substantiated in two very interesting studies from Switzerland.

The first, a survey by F. Verzar and Daniella Gsell, indicated that populations living in the high-altitude Swiss villages had a high intake of dairy fats and a low mortality from cardiovascular disease. The physical activity of these mountain people was continuous and intense.

The second was a detailed study, conducted by Dr. Mayer and Dr. Gsell, of the blood serum cholesterol levels of the Swiss mountain people of one of these villages. They selected Blattendorf, in the southern Swiss Alps, where they showed that, although the villagers' diet consisted of 34 percent dairy fats, their cholesterol was very low by American standards, and even low by comparison to their city-dwelling countrymen. But here is the difference: They have no roads and go everywhere on foot, traveling from an altitude of 4,000 to 8,000 feet and back as part of their daily routine, which indicated that their great physical activity was probably a factor in maintaining the low blood serum cholesterol.

More direct evidence is Dr. Frederick J. Stare's study of several hundred pairs of Irish brothers. One of each pair came to live in Boston, while the other stayed in Ireland. The brothers who came to the United States had two and a half times as many cases of heart disease and heart abnormalities as the brothers who stayed in Ireland and were more active.

Rapid physical deterioration due to weightlessness and inactivity occurred with the astronauts, who had difficulty walking on their return to earth after ten days in space. This is a speeded-up example of what is happening to many in our society today; busy people are free from organic disease, but lose strength, muscle tone, and bone calcium and yet "haven't time to exercise."

Here's how some of us live: In the morning, the hectic businessman gets going with coffee and drags on cigarettes, props himself up with drinks and coffee at lunch and again at dinner time, and ultimately falls into bed in a stupor of narcotic depression from alcohol and nicotine, with an underlying jitteriness from caffeine.

If he's the type who sleeps like a rock, he'll get up in the morning feeling drugged and will need two or three cups of strong coffee to get going and start the cycle again. He may continue to sleep like a rock for a few years, but some day this vicious combination is going to wake him up with the jitters at two to four in the morning because the adrenaline in his system has been stimulated to counteract the narcotics (an alarm reaction of the endocrine glands in an effort to keep us from drugging ourselves to death). He may pace the floor, or he may toss for a while and go back to sleep. But, sooner or later, the idea that he has to get some sleep before that "important meeting" will get him and he'll start taking sleeping pills. Often it starts with the kind easily bought in a drugstore without a prescription. For a while they put him to sleep, but he wakes up feeling logy; so in the morning he takes an extra cup of coffee.

Now the crescendo of the cycle has started; more coffee, pep pills, and then stronger drugs to sleep; additional cocktails at night, which excite more adrenaline in protective response to the narcotic. He is now taking tranquilizers or sleeping pills, or both, in combination with alcohol, which can be lethal. In any event, he may acquire a psychological and physical dependency on stimulants and drugs that is going to be hard to break; so hard that this book may not be able to help unless his doctor has turned him around 180 degrees. However, if we can catch him early enough we can help him because an exercise program and that kind of living are incompatible, psychologically even more than physically. If he is reasonably fit, his body can take a pretty bad beating, but in terms of mental attitude either the exercise or the drug-stimulant cycle will win out and the other side will give in. If, as we hope, the exercise program wins out, the feeling of well-being and happiness is so great he'll lose interest in the drugs, stimulants, and cigarettes.

He may say, ''But I only get about 7 hours sleep now, how can I exercise?'' He would be better off to sleep 6½ hours and do the exercise. However, let's be honest and examine that 7 hours. Is that what he thinks he sleeps? If he was in bed for 8 hours, he probably got more than he thinks. In any case, much of the rest value can be gained from just lying there. The fact that he gets up feeling like the leading character in a Greek tragedy is more often due to the aftereffects of stimulants followed by narcotics than from loss of sleep.

Ultimately, this man must find out the value of an exercise program in combating this cycle. For many people, exercising in the morning is difficult even without working against a hangover, whether from drinks or pills, and no one will accept the added burden consistently. If the determination is there to keep up the program, the restraint and effort to cut down the excesses will start the day and evening before.

It may be a seesaw battle for weeks and months, but when the exercise program wins, it carries enough rewards so that he'll intensely dislike the occasions when he back-slides for reasons of outside pressure or carelessness. No one can completely avoid these slips, but the exercise will build up additional cardiopulmonary reserve, which can handle a period of stress or an occasional shock so that the fit individual will take it in stride.

For a simple illustration of physical stress, take early spring gardening. The tools cause blisters on the hands and the next day unused muscles are stiff and aching. Nature responds in a week or so with calluses as protection and increased muscular strength and endurance. Climb a hill and you puff; but climb hills for a few weeks and nature responds with increased circulation so your lungs and the blood grab more oxygen and the puffing changes into long, even breathing. Or walk and jog a mile a day for a few weeks. Gradually cut out the walking. After a while you'll become less out of breath, it will feel as if pockets down in your back had opened up and a deep breath can pull in twice as much air.

All of these responses are a part of our general and specific adaptation processes. The exercise is the stressor, which sends a mild alarm reaction around the body. This in turn calls for resistance; the body overcompensates, ultimately bringing about the increased endurance and strength.

An excellent example of adaptive response to the environment exists in the high Andes at 17,000 feet. The men work all day in the mines, and then come out and play soccer for an hour or two. They have more oxygen in their blood, and their chests are like barrels, because nature has responded by giving them extra heart and lung capacity to meet these tremendous demands in that very thin air. The body, in its remarkable way, does these things to protect us when conditions become hostile. Safeguards can be built with a little effort, not to the extent of the Andean miners, but sufficient to give us protection in our normal environment.

The widespread ignoring of our need for physical exercise today has caused serious inactivity diseases and malfunctions to the point where 35–50 percent of American youth can't pass the physical and mental tests for military service. You can look around and see young men in their twenties and thirties with growing waistlines, and whose wives have lost their schoolgirl figures. Their youth and strength give them a chance to enjoy life and they are able to stay up late, burning the candle at both ends. But the next day is often a disaster.

A hangover is miserable both from the physical discomfort and the depressing effect of your dissatisfaction with yourself. If you were to substitute 30–45 minutes a day of effort and mild discomfort for a grim day of misery and, besides, get the bonus satisfaction from what you are doing, it seems like a wonderful swap. You can have much more fun in the evening, too, and the next day will remember what happened the night before! There is a sense of really living that comes from such a good exercise program that simply doesn't exist in any other way, not even at the top of some artificial high with its pricking doubt and fear of tomorrow. The true zest for living is strong and clear and untroubled.

A man who had been on this type of program for 1½ years said, "I only wish I had known years ago what I have since found out, and have had fun finding out. I went around for years half alive and did nothing about it, until I had a scare and severe warning. Even then, the light dawned slowly, but with it came an increasing enjoyment of life, although I was beset with many difficulties at the time.''

It has been such a great solution for us, that we would like to bring both the value and the method of this way of life to others to enable them to regain their strength and health. It will also bring a deeply rewarding stability in their personal lives.

3 | The Secret

"Find the boy in the man and then the dream in the boy and that is what your play is."

Dr. George Sheehan

In early Greek mythology, Eros, the beautiful son of Aphrodite and Ares, was god of creation and life. Later, the Greeks gave him dominion over love and play and, very intuitively, represented him as a child, because children know instinctively how to do both.

Waving his little arms and legs in the cradle, the baby grins and looks up at his mother with gurgling laughter. She picks him up and he clings to her warmth with unselfconscious, instinctive love. In a while, he learns to crawl in his play, making little noises as he goes. Getting into everything, he knocks things over and tumbles down the stairs without really hurting himself. The sources and urges to do

these things are deep within the child and are as basic as his
need to touch his mother and be touched and loved in return.

Even thirty years ago no doctor or psychiatrist would
have denied the child's need to play. Today it is recognized
as a lifetime need, which has been lost and buried in most
of us, until even the ability is forgotten. When the Greeks
took the name of their child-god Eros to create the word,
"erotic," it included not only play and pleasure, but also
life, joy, and passion.

When Dr. Sigmund Freud wrote his *Drei Abhandlungen zur Sexualtheorie* (*Three Contributions to the
Sexual Theory*), his approach to sex was so shocking to the
stodgy Victorians that he scared many people away.
Perhaps, like the man who hit the donkey with the club to
get his attention, Freud sought to startle us, so that those
not too stunned would listen to their great advantage. It
wasn't until his later works that his readers really understood that he had restored to the contemporary word
"erotic" its original meaning, which included not only sex,
but also the true Eros spirit of life and meaningful love.

Freud's theory that children, even infants, could
engage in erotic activity was an affront to many people. But
it was only as if he had been pointing to a bud and describing how later it would become a leaf, then part of a
branch, trunk, and tree. It is just the same with a child's
playful activities, such as touching and kissing. They are
motivated solely for the pleasurable sensations they produce, as are the later, more mature expressions of love.
One of Freud's students, Dr. Franz Alexander, pointed out
that an infant's attempts at locomotion were not so much
practical efforts at mastery, but were rather activities done

for sheer enjoyment, which only incidentally led to more adaptive use later on.

A young colt, bounding exuberantly through lush meadow grass, expresses well the enjoyable and frolicking aspect of this phenomenon, which is like Howard Mickel's description of running: "I enjoyed the very feel of my body and its rhythms, the production of sweat, the love affair that developed between myself and Kansas skies, country roads, grass, ponds and wind."

One runner, like Mickel, loved to stride along country lanes, through the woods, and beside the lakes. He even enjoyed the cooling effect of a pouring rain and the wild, rising wind of the storm. Drenched one day by such a summer shower, he came home looking like a spaniel just out of the river. His wife, understanding him, said to their children, "Look at your father, he's happy as a lark!"

We've heard this joy of physical activity likened to the uninhibited pleasures of a child at play. Others say it is similar to the man's euphoria after his run in the rain, as did Charles Hamilton Sorley in "The Song of the Ungirt Runners":

> The rain is on our lips,
> We do not run for prize.
> But the storm the water whips
> And the wave howls to the skies.
> The winds arise and strike it
> And scatter it like sand,
> And we run because we like it
> Through the broad bright land.

On the basis of our personal experience, we have reached the conclusion that this activity is an erotic adventure in the broadest sense of the word and that the most valid and lasting way to regard it is as an end in itself. Although this erotic adventure is derived here from running, it can come equally well from any of the "steady state" sports. We have heard bike riders, distance swimmers, skaters and cross-country skiers go into ecstatic raptures over their activity, just as we have over ours.

Though we are often reminded of the value of prolonged, strenuous exercise to improve our image and health and to promote relaxation, it is difficult for most people to continue in pursuit of these goals alone. The activity only achieves an autonomy when consciousness is altered and realization of the erotic, pleasurable quality is reached. Through perseverance you can become aware of the fundamental emotional need for this activity in response to a natural and healthy impulse.

Vitality is something we need desperately today; we need to explore, to seek fulfillment in quest of worthwhile values. Imagination has infinite dimension, which Carl Jung expressed as a strange paradox that parallels our own theme; even while we reach maturity in one sense, we must retain the ability to draw on the important qualities of childhood. He put it this way:

> The dynamic principle of fantasy is play, a characteristic also of the child, and as such it appears inconsistent with the principle of serious work. But without this playing with fantasy no creative work has ever yet come to birth. The debt we owe to the play of imagination is incalculable.

In the same vein, Dr. Thomas Harris, in *I'm OK, You're OK,* talks about the child within us and the adult within us. While the adult must remain in control to achieve maturity, it must be able to let the child have its day in the sun for fun, laughter, and the joy of living.

When our basic human need for enjoyable play is frustrated by the shallow materialism in our lives, we first feel restless, then a profound boredom and emptiness sets in. This is the classic depression of today.

Man overtaken by this plight is prey to a cycle of Madison Avenue's instant solutions. It's as simple as turning on your radio or TV set; instant gratification and instant relief for everything: aspirin for headaches, laxatives for constipation, tints for gray hair, tranquilizers for nervous tension, coffee or cokes for fatigue; all frustrations, discomforts, or pain eliminated in "seconds"; instant, perennial happiness.

Under this presumption that we can only live our lives constantly free of complaints, the strengthening effect of our reaction to stress is utterly lost, and without it, we become more depressed than ever, the victims of the distorted values of our times.

In this sad condition, we too often forget the art of play and let our grim and serious work attitudes spill over into our games. Sports have a generosity and magnanimity to them when they are done spontaneously and for fun, but competition and professionalism reflect merely an extension of the work attitudes, so that we return on Monday more exhausted mentally and physically than we went home on Friday. If, instead, we were to relearn the art of play, how differently might we relate to others! Then, eventually, we might carry over some of our new and friendly play attitudes into our work.

Activity is a means of relieving everyday tensions, because it removes the nervous residues of our daily existence. In addition, it releases the inhibitions that prevent our joyous and creative feeling from surfacing. It brings sensations of excitement and delight and the opening of an acute perceptivity.

Through activity, the child within liberates us from our oppressive forces, and through imagination reveals to us new vistas that make us more sensitive to nature, beauty, and authentic values. With each fresh truth we reach a new and higher level of consciousness, where we perceive the true erotic experience.

Intolerant of enigma, the human mind searches constantly for absolutes: heaven or hell, love or hate, good or bad, decadent or vital, though it senses simultaneously that reality often lies in between. But here and there man can occasionally grasp a small taste of the absolute, and in this instance he is rewarded by the erotic phenomenon, achieved by working on something he enjoys.

We have journeyed full circle to the philosophy of the ancients in an early Greek myth, which illustrates not only the polarities of what is and what can be, but as well both our belief that man can and must make a choice and our challenge that "lives of quiet desperation" can yield to surging vitality and joy.

> In the beginning, all the Earth was silent, bare and motionless. No grass, nor trees, nor living things enriched its lifeless scene, until Eros emerged and with his arrows pierced the barren ground. Then life, and joy and motion burst forth throughout the Earth.

4 | Motivation

The way to motivation is to find the key that, for you, unlocks the door in the barrier of mental and physical inertia. Opening the door leads to this exciting new life, which is stable and personally secure. Many people merely exist because they either have forgotten or never knew what living really is and, not knowing, there is no limit to their excuses to be inactive.

Even after many years on the program, you may sometimes feel the inertia if you get overtired or a little stale. Once you've really been through the door for any length of time, however, you'll never want to go back. A day or two of rest and you're at it again, because you get hooked on this like nothing else.

Fears of illness or death are not good keys to motivation, but here are several of the better ones.

Self-Image

We all like to look well and feel well, except for one woman, who said, "I don't give a damn how I feel. I just exercise because I want to look my best." Everyone to his own taste. We all want to look trim, and like to wear nice, well-fitting clothes. This is easier with a slim, athletic figure and good carriage than with a figure like a football, or even a basketball, or a figure with a pot belly and a swayback. It's a great feeling to have a stomach that goes in where others go out.

Suggestion

Suggestion is the most powerful aid to motivation that exists. In its simplest form, it is just getting enthused about your program. It helps to do something difficult in a group, be it reducing, exercising, or giving up smoking. It is so much easier if someone else is sweating it out with you and the friendly shoptalk keeps your interest up. Pride and some low-level competition help, but the companionship is most important. An exercise or jogging group of three or four works better than two, as it doesn't fall apart if one can't make it.

The power of suggestion can be stimulated by regular reading in the field. Some recommended books are mentioned in Chapter 8. In addition, subscribe to one of the exercise participation magazines (not the spectator type), in which everybody has a place in the act, regardless of ability. For a beginner or an experienced jogger a subscription to the magazine *Runner's World* (Box 366, Mountain View, California 94040) will do wonders.

If a fine runner lives in your area, try to meet him or her. Ply him with every question you can think of, then let him talk while you keep mental notes. Most experts are glad to do this and give great encouragement to enthusiastic beginners.

Suggestion power can be built by repetitious reminders. Put a sign on your mirror: EXERCISE TODAY. Repeat over and over to yourself: "Must exercise today" and, after your workout, "I will exercise tomorrow." This is particularly effective if you employ a simple form of posthypnotic suggestion by repeating it just before you go to sleep.

Step-by-Step Approach

Take each exercise and each workout as a step in itself. Do the first exercise, then think of the next and do it. Sometimes looking at the summit of the mountain makes faint the heart of the climber, but if he just looks where to put his foot for the next step, he has no problem. He knows he can do it and he does it.

Dr. Warren R. Guild, who practices in the Boston area, has written many books and pamphlets on exercise. He has described how he runs the toughest parts of the Boston Marathon, which he has done most creditably many times. As he approaches the mile-long hill in Newton Lower Falls, he never looks at the top but keeps his eyes riveted on the ground in front of him about 8 feet ahead, and just puts one foot in front of the other and grinds up the slope. Dr. Guild doesn't worry about the famous "Heartbreak Hill," 20 miles out, he breezes up it, but at Kenmore Square (a five-way intersection in the heart of Boston) he has just about a mile to go. At this point a competent marathoner has run 25 miles in 5–6 minutes each. His body, from his feet to his waist, is one solid ache. In the fastest runners it can be real pain. This comes from a combination of the pounding, the terrible effort, and from holding one's body in the same position for such a long time. From then on, Dr. Guild never looks up; he keeps his eyes riveted on the ground and takes each step at a time until he rounds the two final corners and crosses the finish line.

Although it's vitally important to have a definite program of exercise and an objective as to weight, don't set a time limit on reaching that objective, as you might be disappointed or overdo in trying to reach it. Say instead: "My objective is to become fit and, by so doing, lose [for example] 20 pounds. I will take six workouts a week. Each will include exercises first, then walking 2 miles. Later I will walk and jog, and finally jog the whole 2 miles. I will keep a daily record of exercises, times and distances walked and jogged, and weight." (Your weight will go up and down with fluid balance, so work on a weekly average. See Chapter 10).

Some Recommendations

Don't discuss your program with your friends. Your family will have to know about it, and most family members are pretty cooperative once they know you are serious and sticking with it. Some may even join you. There are some great exercising families who exercise together and run together.

Some of your friends will make your life miserable with snide cliches and will try to convince you that you are going to die of a heart attack if you do anything more than sit on your backside watching the Jets or the Mets on TV, smoking, drinking cola, and eating potato chips.

Get ready for the inevitable question: "Why do you run, anyway?" Paul Reese, 59-year-old marathon runner, gave the best answer: "Someone who asks 'What is love?' has never been in love; someone who asks 'Why do you run?' has never run. Only lovers and runners know."

Or this tired old remark: "I don't want to drop dead of a heart attack, so I get my exercise as a pallbearer for my exercising friends." I can best answer this by quoting from Dr. Lawrence E. Lamb's book *Your Heart and How to Live With It:*

> Many a well-intentioned exercise program to improve general health and physical fitness has come to an abrupt end by the improper use of exercise. A military commander may decide that it is time to get all his troops "in shape" and then orders all hands to fall out for an hour of vigorous exercise. Sometimes the middle-aged, overweight, unfit individuals "fall out" permanently, dying with an acute heart attack, causing exercise to be discredited and the program to be discontinued at once. Such events in no way discredit the use of exercise in prevention of heart disease. They merely discredit the uninformed use of exercise by the naive enthusiast.

The rule of thumb to follow to avoid the dangers of overdoing is to increase gradually the amount of exercise above your daily level. Do not expect to accomplish miracles in a short time.

Summary

You must find the key, the open sesame to your motivation. Is your appearance important to you? If you feel poorly and tired, wouldn't you rather feel well all the time? Read up on your type of program. Meet the authors and the experts. Ask them questions and carry the enthusiasm over to others on your own level. Remember, the greatest source of enthusiasm comes from the feeling of well-being that rewards you after you are over the hump. There may be dropouts in the early stages, chiefly among the faddists, but among those who experience the rewards of fitness the proportion who stick with it is very, very high.

Approach your program step by step, and take one step at a time.

Set yourself a weight goal and keep a daily record of your weight. It goes up and down on the fluid balance, but the average comes down eventually (Chapter 10).

Keep a diary of your workout and distances run, with times.

Get your family in the act or get some pals to run with you.

5 | The Action and The Program

"It is the firm conviction of the writer, after a lifetime of study of the subject, that physical fitness is like the trunk of a tree which supports all the rest of the desirable aspects of life: energy, sex life, happiness, and fulfillment to normal expectancy as in youth."

Thomas K. Cureton:
The Physiological Effects of Exercise Programs on Adults

The Need to Exercise

There is an investment consultant in his late thirties, who has a tremendous and lucrative business in New York. As a specialist in certain types of securities, the demands on his time are more than he can supply. His ability to select high-quality securities and to buy them at the right time is unequaled. He has a lovely wife and four children, and leads a life with a strong religious background and an outgoing motivation to help others.

Who is this, the Utopian man? No! He smokes three packs of cigarettes a day, is 35 pounds overweight, and gets so irritable that after 4:00 P.M. he would be better off going home. On the weekends he dashes to the golf course for a round a day. At this point it is probably just as well that he uses a golf cart. In terms of Dr. Cureton's fulfillment, this man is half alive and is typical of the individual for whom this book is written, because, on the basis of the statistics, his chances of a health problem are so great that if he were aware of them he might be frightened enough to do something about it. But no one wants to tell him.

Exercise is one of the principal factors necessary to bring into balance food intake with energy output. It is necessary to keep the blood circulation going so that the various parts of the body, including the brain, keep healthy and do not deteriorate. With our sedentary life, even a young man in his early twenties may begin to get patchy, fatty (atheromatous) thickening in the arteries of his heart and other parts of his body and later calcium deposits may accumulate in their walls. These conditions cause the passages to narrow like water pipes in an old house, thereby reducing the blood supply to the tissues and organs, which suffer from oxygen deficiency as a result.

On the other hand, endurance type exercise over a period of time will build collateral circulation around the heart and throughout the body, at the same time keeping soft and pliable those blood vessels that are as yet undiseased. This takes the strain off the heart and other vital parts of the body and can add years to the person's life.

Exercise is necessary to keep calcium metabolism in balance so that the back doesn't hunch over and the bones don't become brittle (a friend of ours recently broke his ankle stepping off the curb).

It is necessary to balance the frustrations and tensions in our daily life, which cause our glands to pump adrenaline and without compensating activity simply eat us up inside.

With it we can be more stable and keep in a frame of mind that helps us cope with these problems.

Excuses   **1932974**

"I haven't time to exercise" is a frequent refrain because the demands of business conflict with social commitments and the need for time with the family. Often it seems that none of these things gets proper attention. At first, the addition of a 25–30 minute schedule five to six days a week seems impossible and will be very difficult to initiate. But if a program is started and done diligently, it will far more than make up its own time through increased efficiency and productivity; the feeling of well-being will make boring tasks possible to tolerate with a laugh, and work that we like will become a joy.

Popular Misconceptions
About Exercise

"Oh, exercise makes you ravenous and you eat twice as much; you can't reduce by exercising." A well-established program minimizes and lowers appetite. It is true that increased appetites occur in the first two or three weeks, but this disappears as condition improves. Shortly you will begin to eat in balance with your output and will enjoy it more.

"I don't want to get all those huge bulging muscles; what do I need them for? So why exercise?" Those bulging muscles, or hypertrophy, result from certain very special types of exercise handled in a particular way. Quite to the contrary, this program will bring about a firmness of muscle tone and a distinct improvement in appearance, but you won't look like the stereotype of the unlimited class weightlifter. The excessive mass, and even fat, carried by some of these super heavyweights is totally unnecessary. This is demonstrated by the lighter classes of lifters, who handle two and a half times their body weight and have trim and wiry musculature. Olympic champion Dave Wottle is an example of how this works. Dave, who is scarcely known as a weightlifter, can bench-press 180 pounds.

"I never eat lunch (or breakfast), so why don't I lose weight?" Skipping meals is a mistake. The tendency to compensate is so powerful that the person usually ends up by eating more in total. There is also a metabolic problem of "storing" with missed meals. First rule for weight reduction: Eat three meals a day but lighten up all around, particularly the evening meal or, if you can't, step up your activity.

"Oh, she eats like a bird; I've seen her, but she just never loses." Don't you believe it. She is sneaking goodies on the side. The claim of a major metabolic malfunction, "Anything I touch just turns to fat!" is the most overworked excuse in the world.

One man said, as he took a deep drag from his fifteenth cigarette before lunch, "After all, exercise isn't the answer to everything." Of course it isn't. Neither is sex nor food. But without them we wouldn't be around for long.

THE PROGRAM

The broad concept of exercise can be narrowed down into two areas:
1. Recreational exercise, and
2. True fitness exercise, which develops the heart,

blood vessels, and lungs, and limbers and strengthens muscles and joints.

Recreational Exercise

Many games and sports are enjoyable, relaxing, and burn up a few surplus calories, but contribute little to true fitness. Sailing, golf, leisurely tennis, bowling, and a hundred other activities are great fun, but must be classified as recreation, not exercise.

One of their defenders will say: "I played 18 holes of golf in the heat last Sunday, and lost 6 pounds; was I exhausted! You can't tell me that isn't exercise!" However, the 6 pounds were probably 90 percent water and he undoubtedly would have felt better if he had taken some water with a little dissolved salt. He was exhausted because he was in poor shape.

If you do your fitness program, you can be better at your favorite recreation, because it really works. A fitness enthusiast, well along in a good program, has an advantage his fading opponent does not have. The fit golfer on the sixteenth hole in 90° heat will be playing his shots with enthusiasm while his opponent may well lose his concentration through fatigue and slight heat exhaustion. In all games, your coordination, equanimity, and stamina will be outstandingly improved as the result of a fitness program.

True Fitness Exercises: Cardiopulmonary (Aerobic) Exercise, or CPE

From the time of the early Greeks and Romans, each proponent of physical fitness has sponsored his own brand, but only very recently has medical research provided us with factual knowledge as to what true fitness is and should be.

Ken Cooper's *Aerobics* and *New Aerobics* have been described as the jewels in the crown of this research. These books were the first popular presentations of the values of long, sustained (steady state) exercise which, when done over a period of months or years, develops the ability of the cardiopulmonary system to use more oxygen, known as "oxygen uptake."

This subject can get very technical, so let's just say that these cardiopulmonary exercises, or CPE, increase the ability to use oxygen and are the keys to fitness and health. They are: walking–running, swimming, and bike riding, in that order of importance. Walking is put up front because it is at the start of a program, but running is the finest of all and we'll say more about it later.

All of these CPE's, used cautiously and faithfully, will, in time, increase your ability to deliver more oxygen to your tissues until you reach your maximum. The preponderance of current scientific information strongly suggests that you will then be more resistant to many illnesses and may add years to your life.

Calisthenics and Weight Training or General Fitness Exercises (GFE)

Calisthenics and weight training are part of this program because complete fitness requires limberness, flexibility, and strength throughout the entire body as well as in the major joints and muscle groups.

Although an opposing and rapidly diminishing school of thought maintains that only CPE is necessary for total fitness, famous coaches in the United States, Britain,

Yugoslavia, Austria, Germany, and Russia prescribe weight training and calisthenics as a necessary part of the overall training for world class runners as well as other athletes. Certainly the authors' own years of living with these exercises lead us to believe that besides developing limberness and strength they act as an important protective element and supplement to the CPE. Furthermore, the method prescribed herein for doing the GFE has introduced a cardiopulmonary element by doing them within a "Time Frame." Without it there may be a tendency to dawdle, the exercises drag, and you lose the cardiopulmonary effect. However, the Time Frame should be used as a guide, not as a straightjacket. Some days you may not feel as ambitious as others and your time will run over. Don't worry about it. There will be other days when you feel marvelous and you'll complete the exercise in less than the indicated time, which will give you a big lift. When we were working out the schedule, we found that doing the exercises in the Time Frame was more fun and we felt much better after the workouts.

As you improve and can do these exercises faster and with rhythm, you will move smoothly from one to the next. Finally, at the advanced level, you should develop a sustained heart rate of 100–120 for 15 minutes in the GFE without weights and of 110–130 for 26 minutes with weights, which, in addition to the other benefits, provides an additional cardiopulmonary effect as a supplement to the CPE.

The first exercises in each program have been adapted from Dr. Hans Kraus to stretch and limber up your back, the source of the most frequent biological complaint in our society, so that "Oh, my aching back!" has become synonymous with general misery. Then the exercises go on to maintain healthy tissue and adequate strength and flexibility in arms, back, and torso without huge, bulging muscles. This enables you to handle normal life activities such as picking up a child, a heavy suitcase, or moving the baby's crib.

The period to reach your maximum at the advanced level of the GFE has been stretched out over a total of ten months, while the CPE running program only takes five months to reach 2 miles in less than 20 minutes. Since the aerobic program has progressed faster than the calisthenics or weight training, your ability to use oxygen is well ahead of the time when you put the full requirement of effort on the muscles and arteries of your arms and upper back.

Now that you know the real meaning of exercises and fitness, let's get on with the program.

Find a room where you will be undisturbed and you won't disturb others. Open a window slightly, but you don't have to be a fresh air fiend. You need a strong table, a heavy chair, and a blanket folded four to six thicknesses to lie on (on the floor), and one pillow. Select and set up a TV set, radio, or stereo, to your taste. Clothing: shorts, socks, sneakers; for women: bra and panties with a light jersey and shorts. Use clothes you have on hand for now.

Keep track of your resting pulse rate. Lie down for a couple of minutes and take it, as previously described. Write it down and take it every two weeks and keep it on your exercise chart.

Now, when you start, don't try to be a tiger!

It is very important to warm up properly. The first few exercises are designed to do just that. Start the warming-up exercises gently, especially if you have not been exercising lately. Treat yourself kindly until you know how your muscles, tendons, and ligaments react. If you have exercised before, don't let false pride get you with strains and cramps, or worse. There is always another day to do more. Exert slight effort, but no hard effort or strain. Regardless of what you have heard, always exhale during the greatest effort and never, never hold your breath. If you feel queer, dizzy, seasick, or your heart starts to pound, STOP! and check with your doctor.

6 | GFE Without Equipment

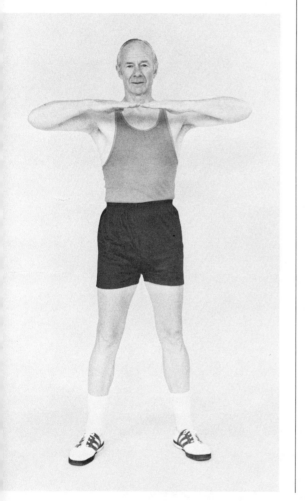

FIRST EXERCISE

ARMS FLINGING

Number of Repetitions
To start (Basic Level): 10
Intermediate Level: 25*

Standing erect, feet apart, raise arms in front of chest.

* For Table of Intermediate and Advanced Levels on all exercises see Page 76.

Number of Repetitions per Workout to Intermediate Level																
Week 1	2	3	4	5	6	7	8	9	10	11	12	13	14	15	16	17
Reps 10	10	12	14	16	18	20	22	24	25	25	25	25	25	25	25	25

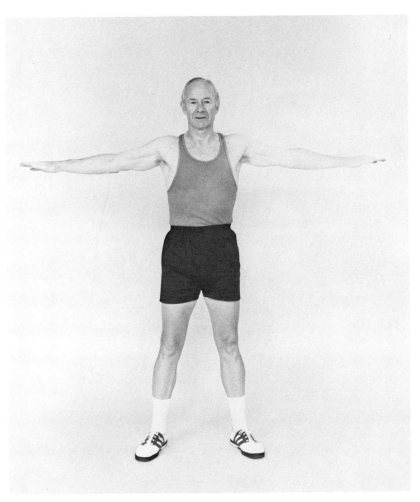

Fling arms to side; exhale as they go out to the side and backwards; inhale as they come in front.

Number of Repetitions per Workout to Advanced Level

Week	18	19	20	21	22	23	24	25	26	27	28	29	30	31	32	33	34	35	36	37	38	39	40	41	42
Reps	27	29	31	33	35	37	39	41	43	45	47	49	50	50	50	50	50	50	50	50	50	50	50	50	50

KNEE EXTENSION AND FLEXION

Number of Repetitions

To start: 5 each side

Intermediate Level: 12 each side

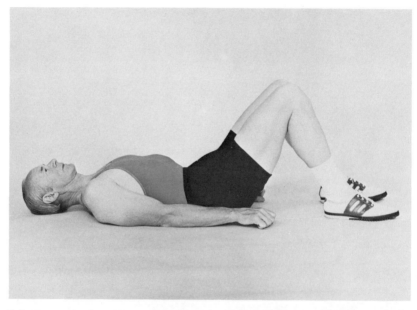

Lie on your back on the blanket; knees bent, hands at sides, palms down.

Number of Repetitions per Workout to Intermediate Level

Week	1	2	3	4	5	6	7	8	9	10	11	12	13	14	15	16	17
Reps	5	5	7	9	11	12	12	12	12	12	12	12	12	12	12	12	12

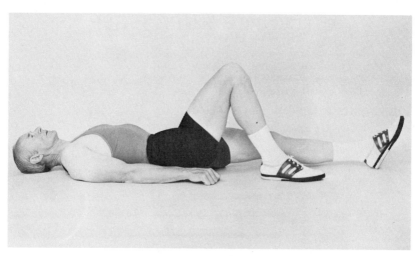

Extend left leg, stretching fully. Inhale when extending leg.

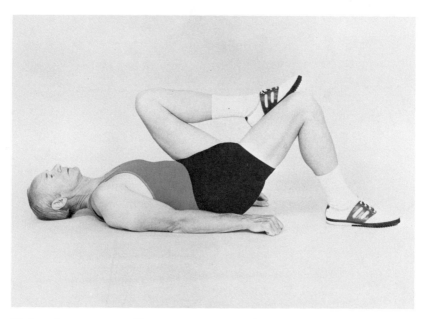

Bring knee up as far as you can without raising head, exhaling as knee comes up. Replace and repeat with right knee.

Number of Repetitions per Workout to Advanced Level

Week	18	19	20	21	22	23	24	25	26	27	28	29	30	31	32	33	34	35	36	37	38	39	40	41	42
Reps	14	16	18	20	20	20	20	20	20	20	20	20	20	20	20	20	20	20	20	20	20	20	20	20	20

ALTERNATE KNEE RAISE

Number of Repetitions

To start: 5 each side
Intermediate Level: 12 each side

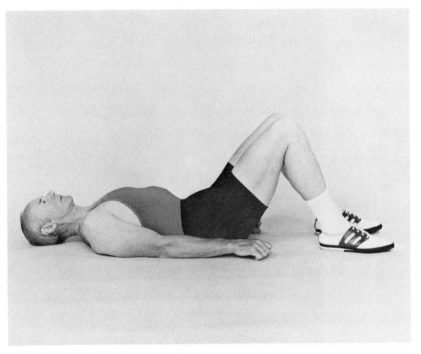

Stay on your back, knees bent.

Number of Repetitions per Workout to Intermediate Level

Week	1	2	3	4	5	6	7	8	9	10	11	12	13	14	15	16	17
Reps	5	5	7	9	11	12	12	12	12	12	12	12	12	12	12	12	12

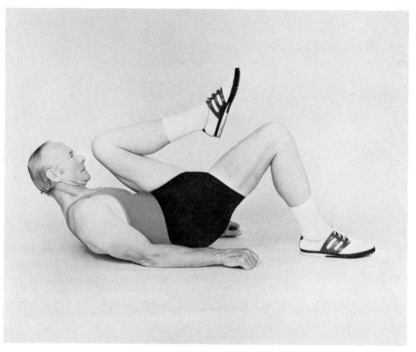

Without extending leg, raise left knee and head at same time. Try to touch nose to knee. Exhale when knee comes up. Inhale when it goes down. Repeat with right knee.

Number of Repetitions per Workout to Advanced Level

Week	18	19	20	21	22	23	24	25	26	27	28	29	30	31	32	33	34	35	36	37	38	39	40	41	42
Reps	14	16	18	20	20	20	20	20	20	20	20	20	20	20	20	20	20	20	20	20	20	20	20	20	20

DOUBLE KNEE RAISE

Number of Repetitions

To start: 5

Intermediate Level: 15

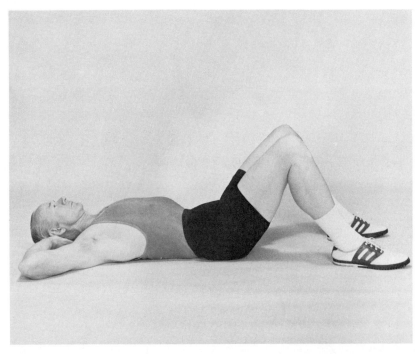

Still on back, place hands behind head.

Number of Repetitions per Workout to Intermediate Level

Week	1	2	3	4	5	6	7	8	9	10	11	12	13	14	15	16	17
Reps	5	5	6	7	8	9	10	11	12	13	14	15	15	15	15	15	15

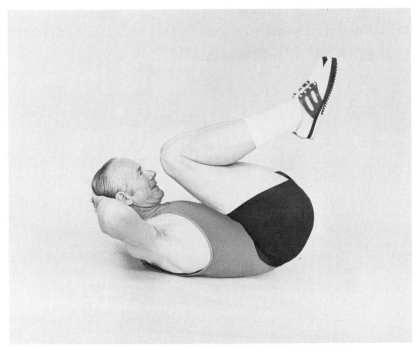

Raise both legs and head as far as you can, exhaling as they come up. Lower legs, inhaling as they go down. If you can't do it, just raise legs slightly.

Number of Repetitions per Workout to Advanced Level

Week	18	19	20	21	22	23	24	25	26	27	28	29	30	31	32	33	34	35	36	37	38	39	40	41	42
Reps	16	17	18	19	20	20	20	20	20	20	20	20	20	20	20	20	20	20	20	20	20	20	20	20	20

HANDS OVERHEAD,
SWINGING TO THE FLOOR

Number of Repetitions

To start: 5 each side
Intermediate Level: 15 each side
Starting position, with feet apart, knees slightly bent and
hips pressed forward, interlace fingers and raise both hands
over head with palms out and up.

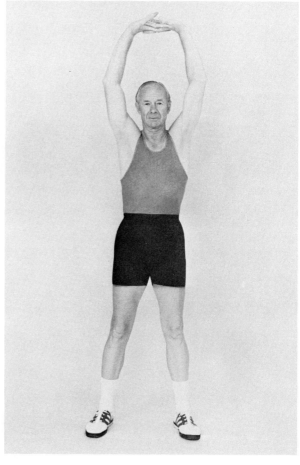

Number of Repetitions per Workout to Intermediate Level

Week	1	2	3	4	5	6	7	8	9	10	11	12	13	14	15	16	17
Reps	5	5	6	7	8	9	10	11	12	13	14	15	15	15	15	15	15

Bending knees, reach down and touch hands to right foot, palms out and down. Inhale going down.

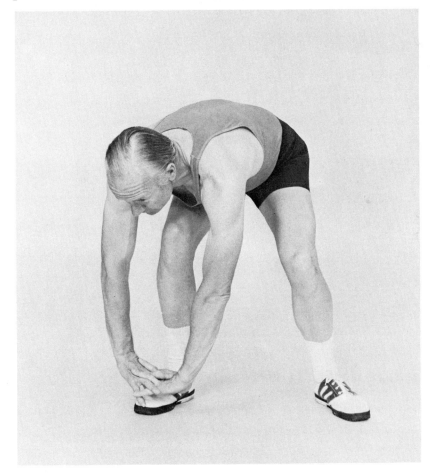

Number of Repetitions per Workout to Advanced Level

eek	18	19	20	21	22	23	24	25	26	27	28	29	30	31	32	33	34	35	36	37	38	39	40	41	42
ps	16	17	18	19	20	20	20	20	20	20	20	20	20	20	20	20	20	20	20	20	20	20	20	20	20

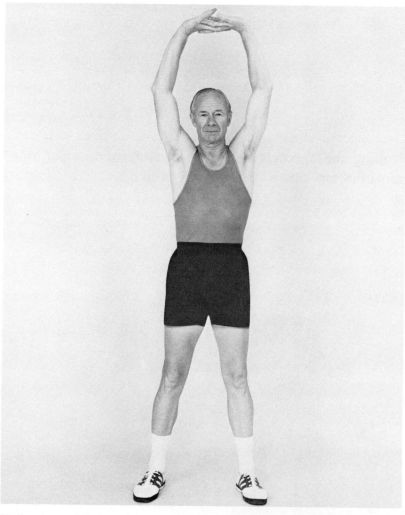

Raise up with hands over head again, exhaling as you come up. This will work better when you get the rhythm because you are exhaling at the point of greatest effort.

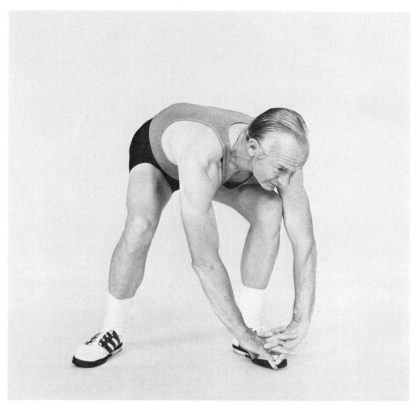

Bend down and touch left foot. When bending down don't let it push your stomach out. Hold it in all the way up and down. Return to starting position and repeat.

BACK EXERCISES*

Number of Repetitions

To start: 2 each
Intermediate Level: 10 each

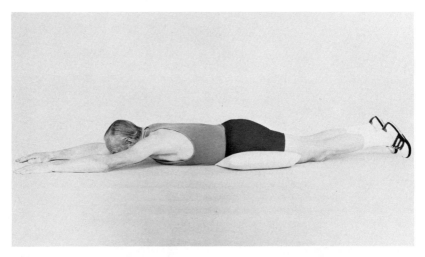

Start. Lie on blanket face down, putting pillow as shown.

* These exercises have been the subject of controversy, chiefly because the exercise is blamed when it is done strenuously by deconditioned people without warming up. However, they are essential exercises for basically healthy people who need to strengthen their back muscles in order to avoid an incident with the back from some normal activity such as bending over to pick something up, lifting a suitcase, etc.

Number of Repetitions per Workout to Intermediate Level

Week	1	2	3	4	5	6	7	8	9	10	11	12	13	14	15	16	17
Reps	2	2	3	4	5	6	7	8	9	10	10	10	10	10	10	10	10

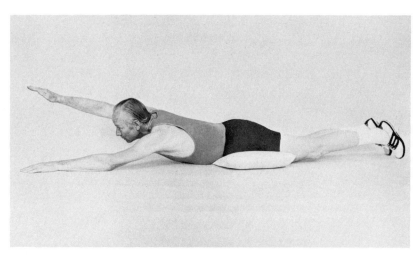

Raise right arm. Exhale coming up; inhale going down in all these exercises.

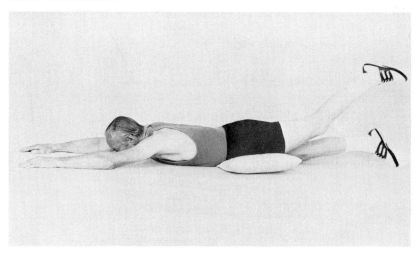

Raise left leg.

Number of Repetitions per Workout to Advanced Level

Week	18	19	20	21	22	23	24	25	26	27	28	29	30	31	32	33	34	35	36	37	38	39	40	41	42
Reps	11	12	13	14	15	15	15	15	15	15	15	15	15	15	15	15	15	15	15	15	15	15	15	15	15

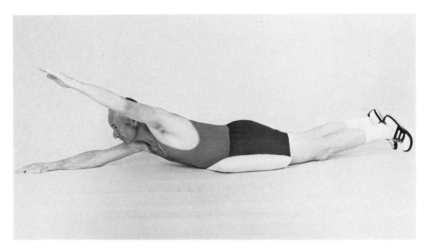

Raise left arm.

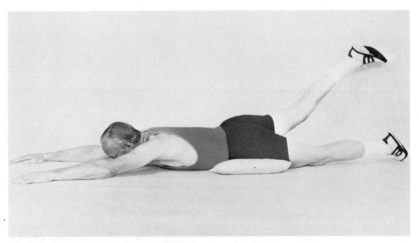

Raise right leg.

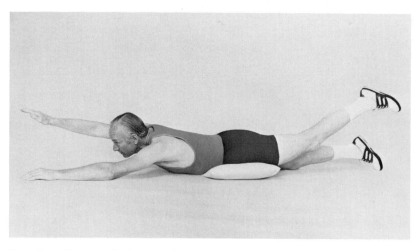

On the diagonal: Raise right arm and left leg, keeping them straight.

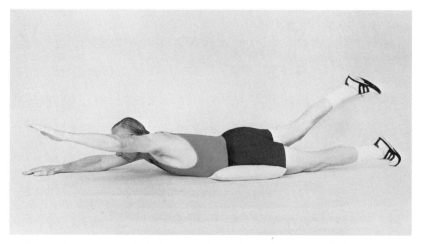

Raise left arm and right leg, keeping them straight.

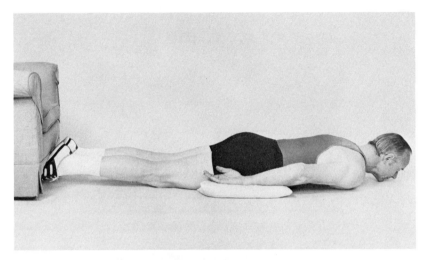

Back raising: Lie with pillow as shown and feet under chair; raise head and shoulders, very slightly at first.

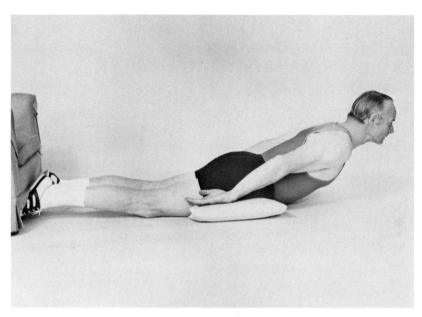

Exhale as you come up; inhale as you go down. This is a difficult exercise. If you have not been exercising, just raise your head at first, then work up to raising head and shoulders.

FIGURE 8

Number of Repetitions

To start: 2 each side
Intermediate Level: 15 each side

Exhale when knees come up; inhale when they go down.

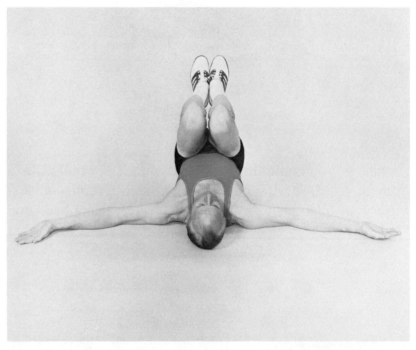

Lie on your back, arms extended on floor, shoulder level.
Palms up. Bend knees up over your chest.

Number of Repetitions per Workout to Intermediate Level

Week	1	2	3	4	5	6	7	8	9	10	11	12	13	14	15	16	17
Reps	2	2	3	4	5	6	7	8	9	10	11	12	13	14	15	15	15

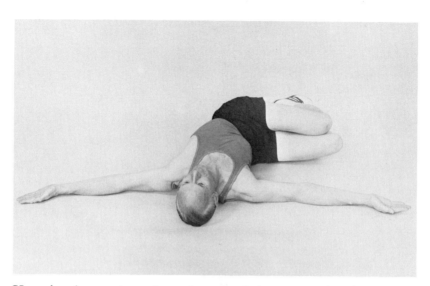

Keeping knees together, drop both knees to the right side, all the way to the floor, and directly out from hips. Keep arms as close to the floor as possible.

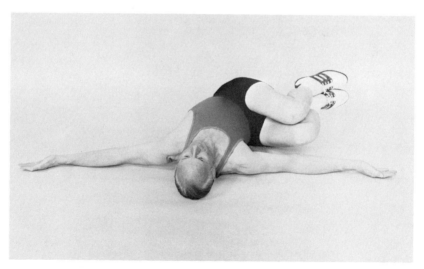

Keeping knees on the floor, pull them up toward elbow. Hold. From this pulled-up position:

Number of Repetitions per Workout to Advanced Level

Week	18	19	20	21	22	23	24	25	26	27	28	29	30	31	32	33	34	35	36	37	38	39	40	41	42
Reps	16	17	18	19	20	21	22	23	24	25	26	27	28	29	30	31	32	33	34	35	36	37	38	39	40

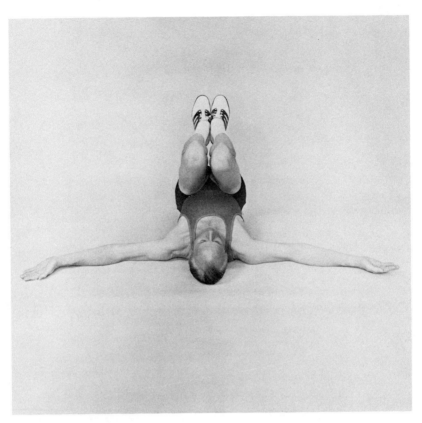

Roll knees back over your chest. Hold.

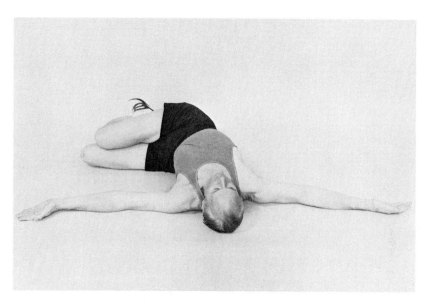

Drop both knees to left side directly out from hips;

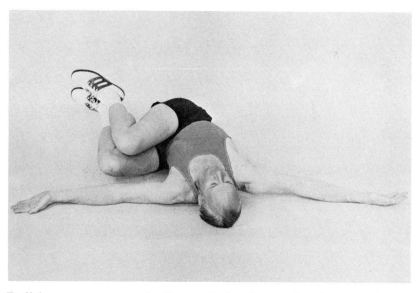

Pull knees up toward elbow. Bring knees back over chest.
Hold.

SIT-UPS

Number of Repetitions

To start: 5
Intermediate Level: 20 with hands behind head

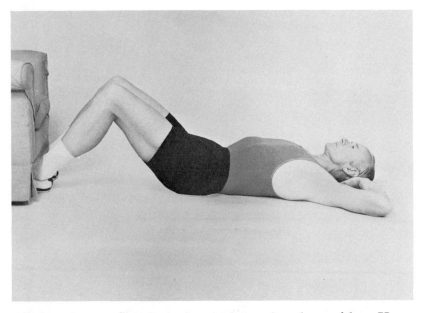

Anchor feet under chair, knees bent, hands at sides. Keep
back flat on floor, never arched.

Number of Repetitions per Workout to Intermediate Level

Week	1	2	3	4	5	6	7	8	9	10	11	12	13	14	15	16	17
Reps	5	5	6	7	8	9	10	11	12	13	14	15	15	15	15	15	15

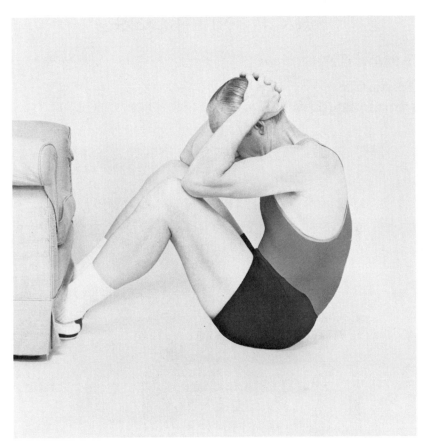

Sit up with a rolling motion so back is rounded all the way up. Exhale coming up. If you can't do it, push with your hands to help. Repeat. Later you can do it without the push. Then, fold arms on chest. Much later you can place hands behind head as shown in picture. Inhale going down.

Number of Repetitions per Workout to Advanced Level

Week	18	19	20	21	22	23	24	25	26	27	28	29	30	31	32	33	34	35	36	37	38	39	40	41	42
Reps	16	17	18	19	20	21	22	23	24	25	25	25	25	25	25	25	25	25	25	25	25	25	25	25	25

HALF KNEE BENDS

Number of Repetitions

To start: 5
Intermediate Level: 15

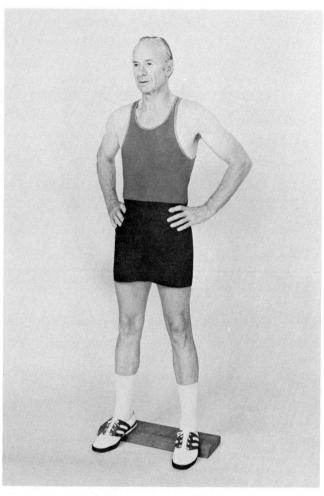

Standing position (on beveled 1½-inch board); hands on hips. Keep feet parallel, 8 inches apart.

Number of Repetitions per Workout to Intermediate Level

Week	1	2	3	4	5	6	7	8	9	10	11	12	13	14	15	16	17
Reps	5	5	6	7	8	9	10	11	12	13	14	15	15	15	15	15	15

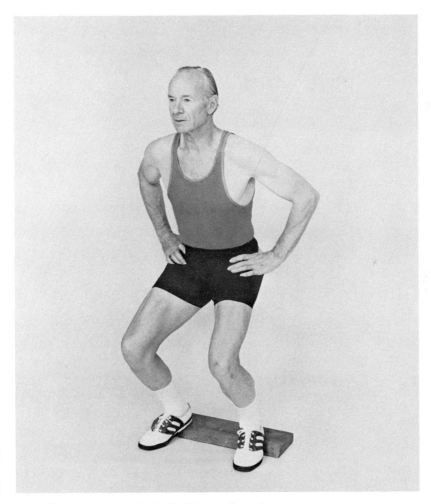

Do half knee bend, inhaling going down.

Number of Repetitions per Workout to Advanced Level

ek	18	19	20	21	22	23	24	25	26	27	28	29	30	31	32	33	34	35	36	37	38	39	40	41	42
ps	16	17	18	19	20	21	22	23	24	25	25	25	25	25	25	25	25	25	25	25	25	25	25	25	25

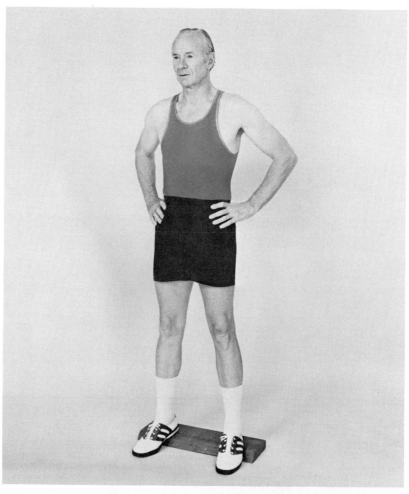

Return to standing position. Exhale coming up.

EASY PULL-UPS

Number of Repetitions

To start: 5

Intermediate Level: 15

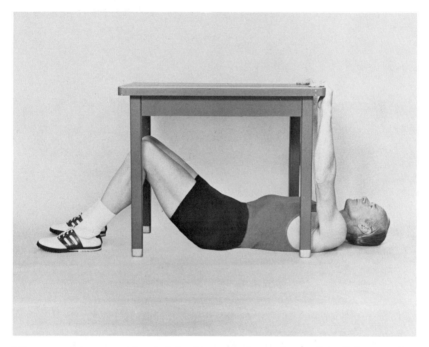

First make sure the table is strong and won't slide or tip.
Then hang under table with knees bent. The more they are
bent, the easier it will be. Be sure arms are fully extended.

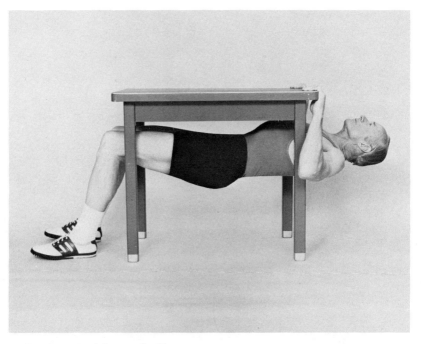

Pull up to table, exhaling as you come up.

Number of Repetitions per Workout to Intermediate Level																
Week	1	2	3	4	5	6	7	8	9	10	11	12	13	14	15	16	17
Reps	5	5	6	7	8	9	10	11	12	13	14	15	15	15	15	15	15

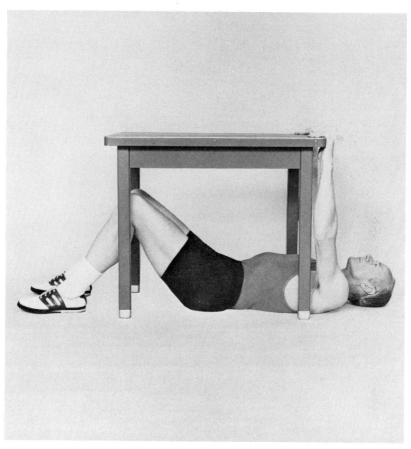

Lower yourself slowly until your arms are fully extended. Inhale as you go down. As the exercise becomes easier, gradually straighten your legs.

Number of Repetitions per Workout to Advanced Level

Week	18	19	20	21	22	23	24	25	26	27	28	29	30	31	32	33	34	35	36	37	38	39	40	41	42
Reps	16	17	18	19	20	20	20	20	20	20	20	20	20	20	20	20	20	20	20	20	20	20	20	20	20

PUSH-UPS

Number of Repetitions

To start: 5
Intermediate Level: 15 on floor

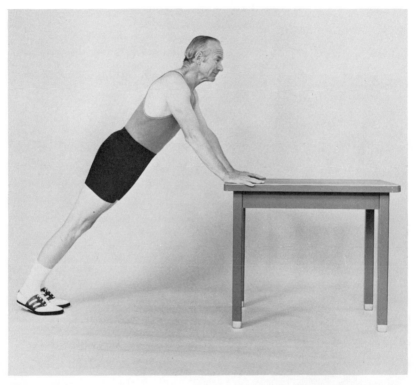

Having made sure your table is strong and won't slide or tip, lean forward with your back straight and place your hands on it.

Number of Repetitions per Workout to Intermediate Level																
Week 1	2	3	4	5	6	7	8	9	10	11	12	13	14	15	16	17
Reps 5	5	6	7	8	9	10	11	12	13	14	15	15	15	15	15	15

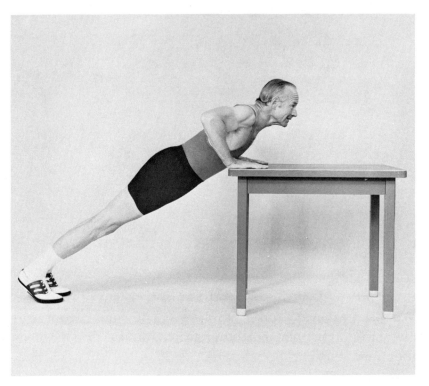

Do a push-up at whatever angle you can comfortably. Inhale going down.

Number of Repetitions per Workout to Advanced Level

eek	18	19	20	21	22	23	24	25	26	27	28	29	30	31	32	33	34	35	36	37	38	39	40	41	42
ps	16	17	18	19	20	20	20	20	20	20	20	20	20	20	20	20	20	20	20	20	20	20	20	20	20

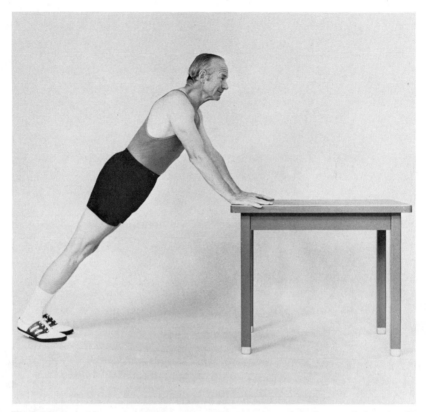

Exhale coming up. Be sure to keep your back straight at all times and look at the wall in front of you, not at the floor. When you can do ten repetitions easily, move your feet away from the table. The ultimate is to do them on the floor touching your chest each time.

NOW REPEAT FIRST EXERCISE

Keep the above schedule at the starting number of repetitions as follows:

Through Age 39: For 2 weeks. Then, if you are not stiff and are feeling fine, add two repetitions per week for exercises 1–3 and one repetition for exercises 4–11 until Intermediate Level is reached.

Age 40–55: Keep the original schedule for 3 weeks and add two per week of exercises 1–3 and one per week of exercises 4–11.

Age 56 and up: Keep original schedule for 4 weeks and add two per week of exercises 1–3 and one per week of exercises 4–11, providing no stiffness or other difficulties develop. However, the individual in this bracket has to use common sense and slack off if it doesn't feel right, since at this point in his career he will probably have arrived at the age of discretion.

Use the Time Frame on page 77 for all of these brackets.

INTERMEDIATE AND ADVANCED LEVELS FOR GFE WITHOUT WEIGHTS

The Intermediate Level is the lowest level at which you can keep sensibly fi
The Advanced Level is the recommended level for good, sound fitness withou
becoming a fiend on the subject, using as a guide the Time Frame chart o
page 77.

No.	Exercise	Intermediate Level No. of Reps	Times Per Week	Advanced Level No. of Reps	Time Per Wee
1.	Arms Flinging	25	5	50	4
2.	Knee Extension and Flexion	12 each side	5	20 each side	4
3.	Alternate Knee Raise	12 each side	5	20 each side	4
4.	Double Knee Raise	15	5	20	4
5.	Hands Overhead, Swinging to the Floor	15 each side	5	20 each side	4
6.	Back Exercises	10 each	5	15 each	4
7.	Figure 8	15 each side	5	40 each side	4
8.	Sit-ups	20 with hands behind head	5	40 with hands behind head	4
9.	Half Knee Bends	15	5	25	4
10.	Easy Pull-Ups	15	5	20	4
11.	Push-Ups	15 on floor	5	20 on floor	4
	Repeat Exercise 1	25	5	50	4

TIME FRAME

Time in Minutes

Week	Through Age 39	Age 40–55	Age 56 and up
1	6	7	8
2	5½	6½	7½
3	5	6	7
4	5½	6	6½
5	6	6½	7
6	6½	7	7½
7	7	7½	8
8	7½	8	8½
9	8	8½	9
10	8½	9	9½
11	9	9½	10
12	9½	10	10½
13	10	10½	11
14	10	11	11½
15	10	11	12
16	10½	11	12
17 (Intermediate Level)	10½	11½	12
18	10½	11½	12½
19	11	12	13
20	11½	12½	13½
21	11½	12½	13½
22	11½	12½	13½
23	11	12	13
24	10½	11½	12½
25*	10	11	12
42 and up (Advanced Level)	15	16	17

* Use a steady progression from 25th week up to Advanced Level.

7 | GFE With Barbell and Dumbbell Weight Training

In the previous program of general fitness exercises, the workout has been reduced to the minimum as far as space, inconvenience, and expense are concerned. However, if you are more ambitious and want to get the added benefits of weight training, a pair of dumbbells and a barbell, which should have weights to put on or take off, will add interest and fun to the workout. Weight training within the prescribed Time Frame will make a supplementary contribution to cardiopulmonary endurance as well as develop increased local blood supply, strength, and limberness of muscles and joints.

Alternate General Fitness
Exercises Using Dumbbells
and Barbell

The type of equipment described below is available in most sporting-goods stores. Be sure to get the type that permits you to add and deduct weights.

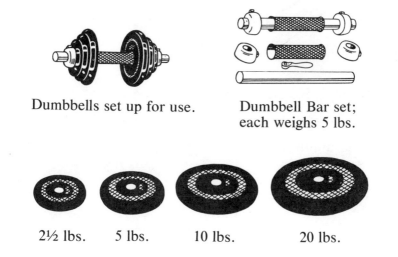

Dumbbells set up for use.   Dumbbell Bar set;
                                   each weighs 5 lbs.

2½ lbs.   5 lbs.   10 lbs.   20 lbs.

   If you have to make a choice between the dumbbells and the barbell, pick the barbell, as most of the exercises are done with it. Also needed are the chair, the pillow or folded towel, and blanket for the floor.

   Start with the barbell alone, no weights attached. However, if it has a chrome sleeve, lock the sleeve in the center with the two interior locking collars. One of our barbells alone, a 5-foot "Bur" with sleeve and interior and exterior locking collars, weighs 19.3 lbs. The sleeve is marked with an etched design to indicate the center and two symmetrically placed hand holds so that the bar can be grasped and raised in balance.

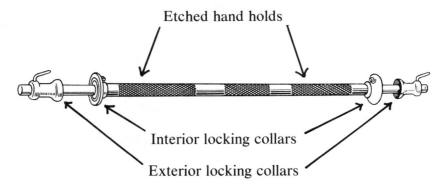

Etched hand holds

Interior locking collars

Exterior locking collars

Bar with sleeve and locking collars

If for any reason this is too heavy, start these exercises with the dumbbell handles, which should weigh no more than 5 lbs. each.

GFE WITH WEIGHT TRAINING

To start this program turn back to pages 42 through 63. Do Exercises 1–7, which are the same in both GFE programs. They will warm you up and get you all set for the eighth exercise, which follows.

For Table of Intermediate and Advanced Levels for GFE with weight training, see pages 114–117, and for the Time Frame, see page 118.

SIT-UPS

Number of Repetitions

To start: 5

Intermediate Level: 20 with hands behind head

This exercise is exactly the same as in General Fitness Exercise 8, and up to the point where you can do it with your hands behind your head to the intermediate level of 20×, it remains the same. When this number of repetitions is completely comfortable, take a 5-pound dumbbell handle and hold it in both hands behind your head. Remember, make a reasonable effort; do not strain! If you can do five

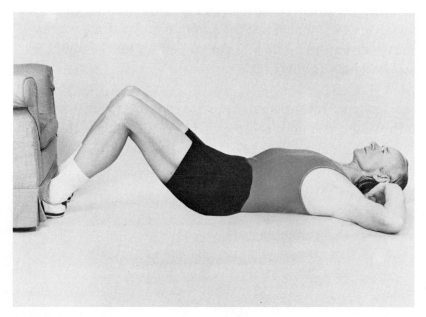

Anchor feet under chair, knees bent. Sit up with a rolling motion so back is rounded all the way up. Exhale coming up; inhale going down.

sit-ups, add one or two a week until you are back to 20. The objective is to add weight gradually until the dumbbell is up to 15 lbs. (maximum). Since the lowest weights are 2½ lbs. each, you should add the locking devices first, and then add two 2½-pound weights without the locking devices. It is quite simple to just hold them in place. This should make the steps 5 lbs. to 7 lbs. to 10 lbs. to 12 lbs. and, finally, to 15 lbs. When you are at 20× with 15 lbs., you are halfway to the advanced level, which is 40× with 15 lbs. Add reps at the rate of one or two a week. If at any point it gets too difficult, split your reps into two sets of 12–15× each, with a 30–60 second rest in between. Then work gradually up to 40× by adding reps to the first set.

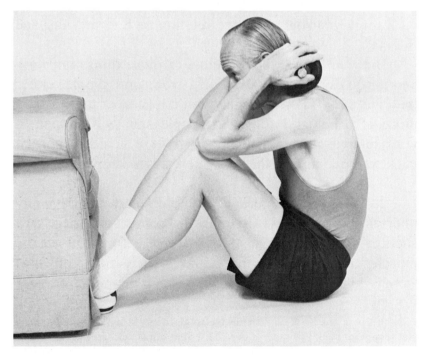

Back should be rounded.

LIFTS

WARNING!
This warning with the lift exercises is from two points of view:
1. If you don't do them.
2. If you do do them.

1. If you decide not to do the lifts and the other back exercises, No. 6 and 11, you, like most Americans, will run the high risk of becoming subject to one of the most common complaints, the aching back. Furthermore, you better not load the suitcases in the trunk of the car* for your vacation trip, move a typewriter for that pretty secretary in the office (an old electric weighs 48 pounds), or pick up a three-year-old child to give him or her an "airplane ride."

But you'll probably do most of these things anyway, and if you don't keep your back strong and supple, either they will get you or some day you'll lean over to pick up a piece of paper and something unpleasant will happen in your lumbar region. So, if you have a healthy, normal back, we recommend the back exercises to keep it that way.

2. On the other hand, if you do do them and have any undisclosed weakness or injury in your back, there is a slight risk that you may strain yourself before you get the muscles built up. The bar alone with which you start weighs less than the heavy suitcase, typewriter, or your

---

* The lift over the back partition in the trunk of any American sedan puts a strain on your back that is ten times the weight of the suitcase. No backbone or disk alone and unsupported can stand it, but strong back and stomach muscles form a powerful column that can carry the weight properly.

child, and by the ninth exercise you should be well warmed up, which you are not when you suddenly grab one of these other objects.

In the following schedule you have four months in which to strengthen your back before adding weight. Follow the schedule intelligently. If the bar is too heavy to start, use the dumbbell handles. If the progression of repetitions (reps) or added weight is too tough, stay at the same level or go back to a lower one for a couple of extra weeks.

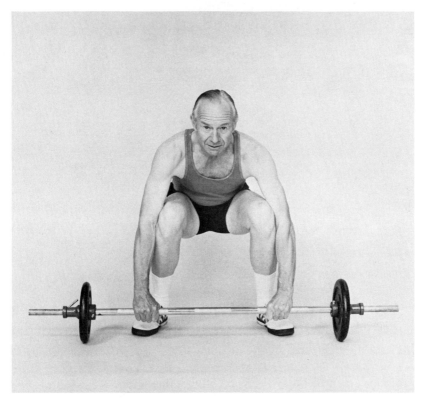

Now, place the bar with sleeve and locking collars on the floor in front of you, and bending your knees lean forward and grasp it in balance, palms facing you.

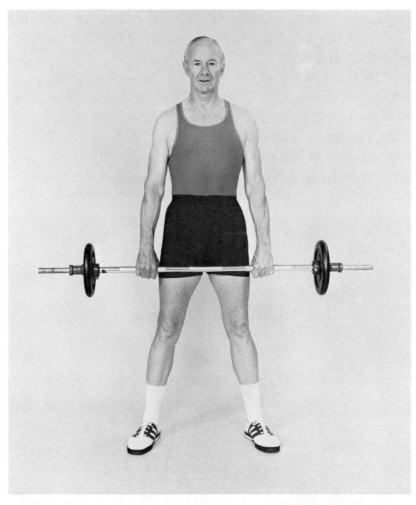

Then, stand up to the correct posture position, keeping your knees bent and under you so they take the brunt of the lift. Exhale as you come up.

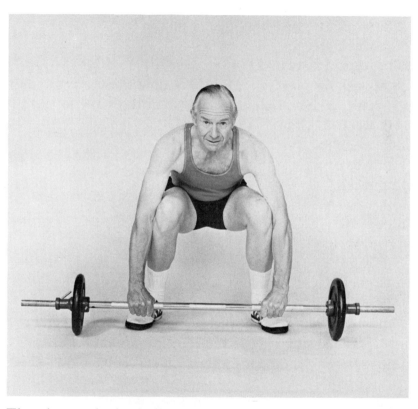

Then lower the barbell to the floor with knees bent and repeat. Inhale going down.

Repeat.

Number of Repetitions:

To start: 3×
 1st 2 weeks 3×
 3rd week 4×
 4th week 5×
 5th week 3×, rest (less than 1 min.), 3×
 6th week 4×, rest, 4×
 7th week 5×, rest, 5×
 8th week 6×, rest, 6× (If at any time these are too diffi-
     cult, take an extra week or so at the same level.)
 9th week 7×, rest, 7×
 10th week 8×, rest, 8×
 11th week 6×, rest, 6×, rest, 6×
 12th week 7×, rest, 7×, rest, 7×
 13th week 8×, rest, 8×, rest, 8×
 14th week add 2½ lbs. at each end of bar, 8×, rest, 8×,
     rest, 8×
 15th week 8×, rest, 8×, rest, 8× (In these weeks start re-
     ducing rest period to 30 seconds or less.)
 16th week 8×, rest, 8×, rest, 8×
 17th week 8×, rest, 8×, rest, 8× (With 10–20 second rest
     periods, this is your Intermediate Level.)
 18th–21st week add 5 lbs. (2½ each end of bar), do 3 sets 8
     reps
 22nd–25th week add 5 lbs., do 3 sets 8 reps
 26th–29th week add 5 lbs., do 3 sets 8 reps
 30th–33rd week add 5 lbs., do 3 sets 8 reps
 34th–37th week add 5 lbs., do 3 sets 8 reps

Bar now weighs 50 lbs. Consult Intermediate and Advanced
Level table on pages 114–115 before adding more weight,
then go to your Advanced Level by adding 5 lbs. every four
weeks. (It is recommended that the maximum weight of the
barbell should be one-half your weight or 90 lbs., whichever
is less.)

HALF-KNEE BENDS

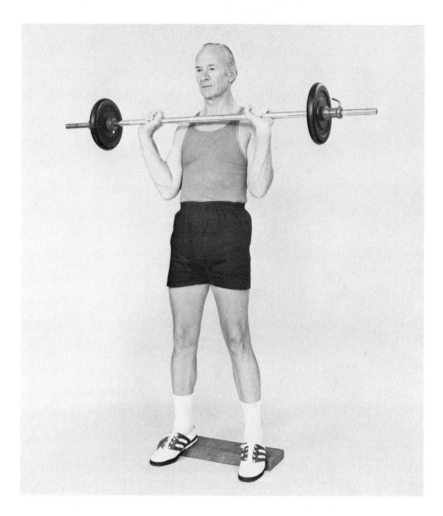

Raise the barbell as in Ninth Exercise, palms facing you; then raise the barbell to your chest, arms bent. Exhale coming up.

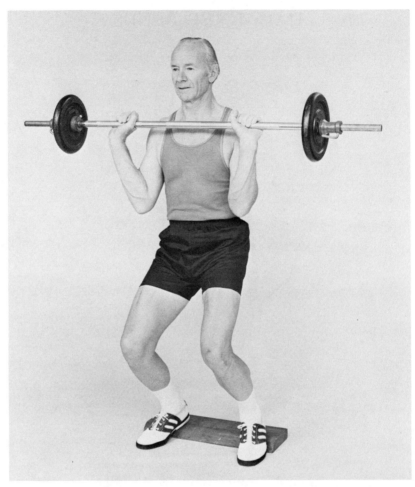

In this position do half-knee bends, feet parallel 8 to 10 inches apart. Inhale going down. Repeat. Replace barbell on floor. Skiers with flexible ankles won't need it, but for others it helps to place a 1½-inch board under the heels while doing this exercise.

Number of Repetitions

To start: 3×

Intermediate Level is reached on same schedule as in Ninth Exercise, which is summarized as follows:

1st 2 weeks 3×
3rd week 4×
4th week 5×
5th week 3×, rest (less than 1 min.), 3×
6th week 4×, rest, 4×
7th week 5×, rest, 5×
8th week 6×, rest, 6×
9th week 7×, rest, 7×
10th week 8×, rest, 8×
11th week 6×, rest, 6×, rest, 6×
12th week 7×, rest, 7×, rest, 7×
13th week 8×, rest, 8×, rest, 8×
14th–17th week add 5 lbs., do 3 sets 8 reps (In these weeks start reducing rest period to 30 seconds or less and in 17th week, with a 10–20 second rest period, this is your Intermediate Level.)
18th–21st week add 5 lbs., do 3 sets 8 reps
22nd–25th week add 5 lbs., do 3 sets 8 reps
26th–29th week add 5 lbs., do 3 sets 8 reps
30th–33rd week add 5 lbs., do 3 sets 8 reps
34th–37th week add 5 lbs., do 3 sets 8 reps

Bar now weighs 50 lbs. Consult Intermediate and Advanced Level table on pages 114–115 before adding more weight, then go to your Advanced Level by adding 5 lbs. every four weeks. (It is recommended that the maximum weight of the barbell should be one-half your weight or 90 lbs., whichever is less.)

LIFT FROM FLOOR TO OVERHEAD (MODIFIED CLEAN AND PRESS)

For the Eleventh and Twelfth Exercises you should check your ceiling height. The needed clearance can be measured by standing, feet together, and extending arms straight up. If your fingertips clear, or just touch, you are about right with the 20-pound weights on the barbell. Putting your feet farther apart will give you a little additional clearance.

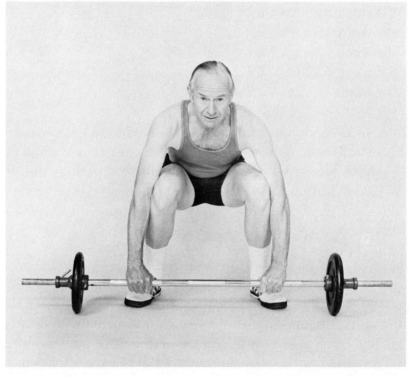

Stand with feet fairly far apart, facing barbell. Reach down. With knees well bent, grasp it in balance with hands apart the width of your shoulders, palms facing toward your feet.

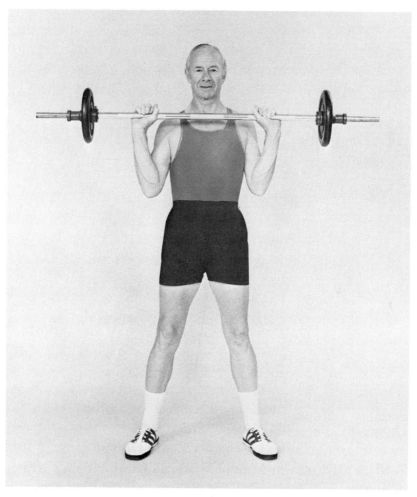

In one smooth movement, bring the barbell up as you stand up, so that it is across your upper chest. Exhale when raising bar.

If you need it, inhale quickly in this position.

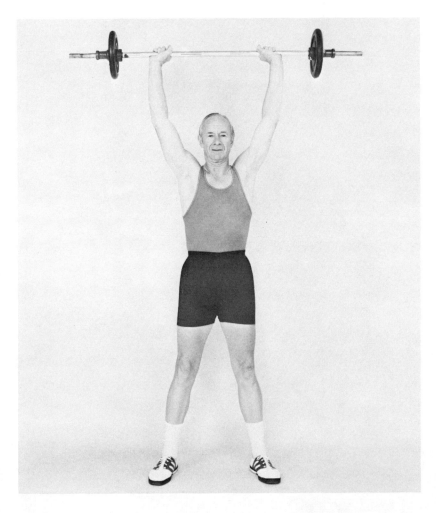

Then press barbell overhead until arms are straight. In the last motion, keep knees slightly bent and hips pressed forward. This takes any undue strain off your back, which should be flat at all times (never arched). Exhale pressing the barbell overhead. Lower barbell and repeat motion. (The purpose of this exercise is to strengthen back, shoulders, and arms, without injury. The instructions are not designed to make you a weight lifter.)

Number of Repetitions

To start: 3×

Intermediate Level is reached on the following schedule:

 1st 2 weeks 3×
 3rd week 4×
 4th week 5×
 5th week 3×, rest (less than 1 min.), 3×
 6th week 4×, rest, 4×
 7th week 5×, rest, 5×
 8th week 6×, rest, 6×
 9th week 7×, rest, 7×
10th week 8×, rest, 8×
11th week 6×, rest, 6×, rest, 6×
12th week 7×, rest, 7×, rest, 7×
13th week 8×, rest, 8×, rest, 8×
14th–17th week add 5 lbs., do 3 sets 8 reps (In these weeks
     start reducing rest period to 30 seconds or less and in
     17th week, with 10–20 second rest period, this is your
     Intermediate Level.)
18th–21st week add 5 lbs., do 3 sets 8 reps
22nd–25th week add 5 lbs., do 3 sets 8 reps
26th–29th week add 5 lbs., do 3 sets 8 reps
30th–33rd week add 5 lbs., do 3 sets 8 reps
34th–37th week add 5 lbs., do 3 sets 8 reps

Bar now weighs 50 lbs. Consult Intermediate and Advanced Level table on pages 116–117 before adding more weight, then go to your Advanced Level by adding 5 lbs. every four weeks. (It is recommended that the maximum weight of the barbell should be one-third your weight.)

OVERHEAD PRESS (MILITARY PRESS)

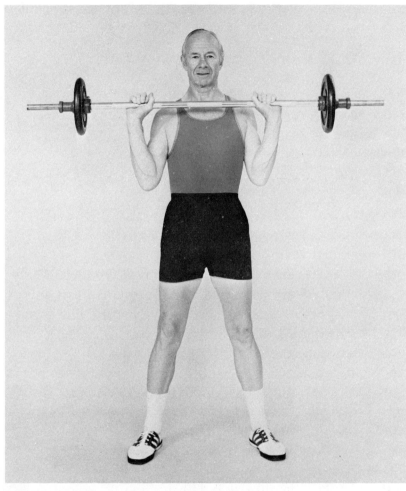

Lift barbell from floor to chest position.

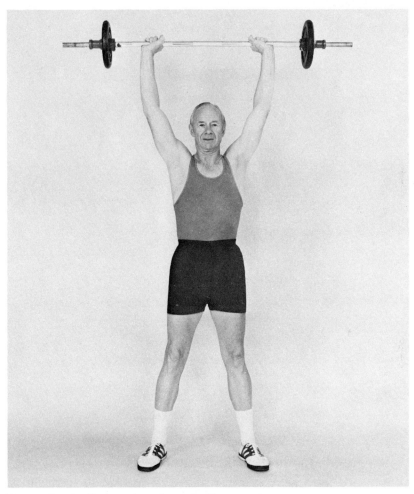

Press barbell overhead, exhaling as it goes up.

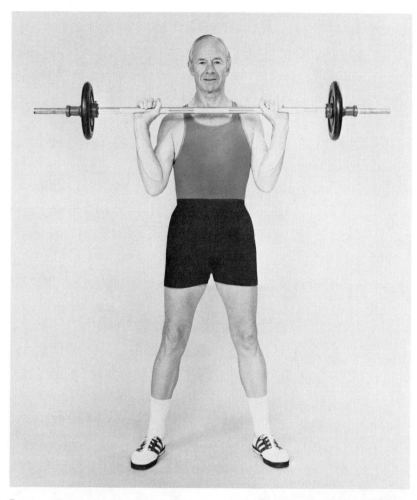

Lower barbell to chest position, inhaling as it comes down.
Repeat press correct number of times and lower barbell to
floor.

Number of Repetitions

To start: 3×

Intermediate Level is reached on the following schedule:

  1st 2 weeks 3×
  3rd week 4×
  4th week 5×
  5th week 3×, rest (less than 1 min.) 3×
  6th week 4×, rest, 4×
  7th week 5×, rest, 5×
  8th week 6×, rest, 6×
  9th week 7×, rest, 7×
  10th week 8×, rest, 8×
  11th week 6×, rest, 6×, rest, 6×
  12th week 7×, rest, 7×, rest, 7×
  13th week 8×, rest, 8×, rest, 8×
  14th–17th week add 5 lbs., do 3 sets 8 reps (In these weeks
      start reducing rest period to 30 seconds or less and in
      17th week, with a 10–20 second rest period, this is
      your Intermediate Level.)
  18th–21st week add 5 lbs., do 3 sets 8 reps
  22nd–25th week add 5 lbs., do 3 sets 8 reps
  26th–29th week add 5 lbs., do 3 sets 8 reps
  30th–33rd week add 5 lbs., do 3 sets 8 reps
  34th–37th week add 5 lbs., do 3 sets 8 reps

Bar now weighs 50 lbs. Consult Intermediate and Advanced Level table on pages 116–117 before adding more weights, then go to your Advanced Level by adding 5 lbs. every four weeks. (It is recommended that the maximum weight of the barbell should be one-third your weight.)

BICEPS CURL

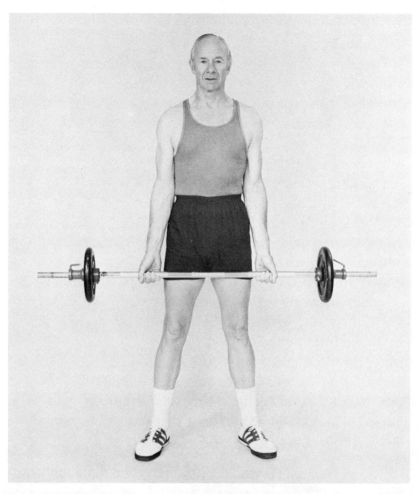

Standing up straight, grasp barbell at shoulder width, palms facing away from legs.

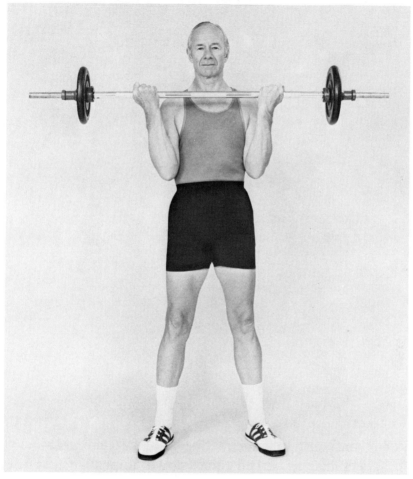

Bring barbell up to shoulder height, exhaling as it comes up.

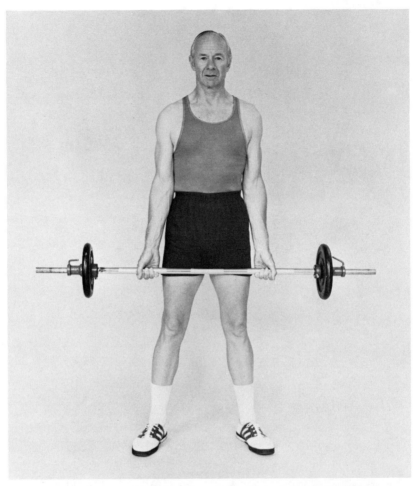

Lower barbell making sure that arms become absolutely straight. Inhale as barbell comes down. Repeat curl correct number of times and lower barbell to floor.

Number of Repetitions

To start: 3×
Intermediate Level is reached on the following schedule:

  1st 2 weeks 3×
3rd week 4×
4th week 5×
5th week 3×, rest (less than 1 min.), 3×
6th week 4×, rest, 4×
7th week 5×, rest, 5×
8th week 6×, rest, 6×
  9th week 7×, rest, 7×
10th week 8×, rest, 8×
11th week 6×, rest, 6×, rest, 6×
12th week 7×, rest, 7×, rest, 7×
13th week 8×, rest, 8×, rest, 8×
14th–17th week add 5 lbs., do 3 sets 8 reps (in these weeks
    start reducing rest period to 30 seconds or less and in
    17th week, with a 10–20 second rest period, this is
    your Intermediate Level.)
18th–21st week add 5 lbs., do 3 sets 8 reps
22nd–25th week add 5 lbs., do 3 sets 8 reps
26th–29th week add 5 lbs., do 3 sets 8 reps
30th–33rd week add 5 lbs., do 3 sets 8 reps
34th–37th week add 5 lbs., do 3 sets 8 reps

Bar now weighs 50 lbs. Consult Intermediate and Advanced Level Table on pages 116–117 before adding more weight, then go to your Advanced Level by adding 5 lbs. every four weeks. (It is recommended that the maximum weight of the barbell should be one-fourth of your weight.)

BENCH PRESS

This is an excellent exercise for strengthening the chest (pectoral) muscles and the shoulders. It requires a piece of equipment, a bench press, which is useful for other exercises, and can be purchased or built inexpensively as shown on page 109.

Bench Press with barbell in the rack.

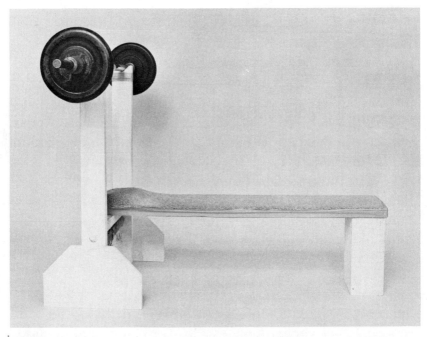

When you have your bench, place the bar, without weights, on the rack provided for it.

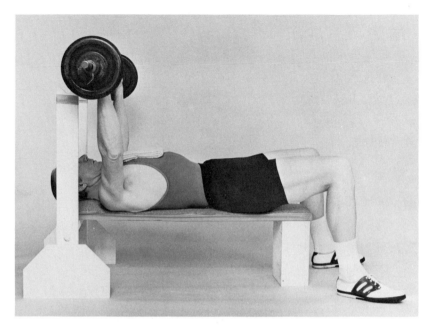

Lie on the bench and take a wide hand hold, out to the interior collars, and lift it off the rack, arms extended.

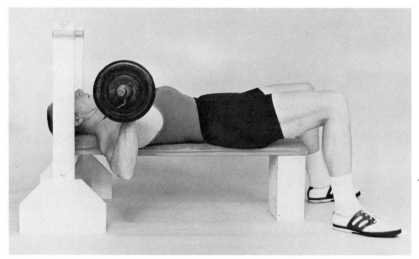

Then lower the bar to your chest inhaling, arms flexed.

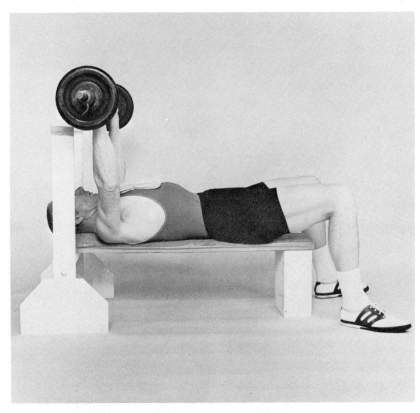

Press up to arms length, exhaling. If you have been doing push-ups, the weight of the bar alone may be too light. If so, add weight until pressing the bar is a reasonable effort without strain. Since the bar should be lowered all the way to the chest to get the maximum extension of the pectoral muscles, it is a good idea to place a pad or folded towel on your chest to prevent discomfort.

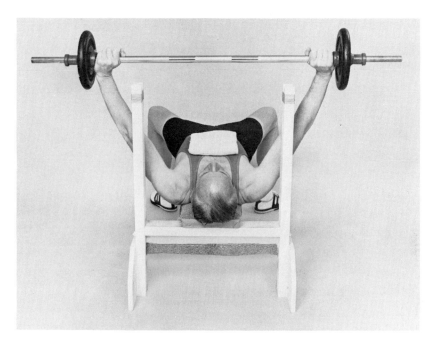

End view, barbell removed from rack, arms extended.

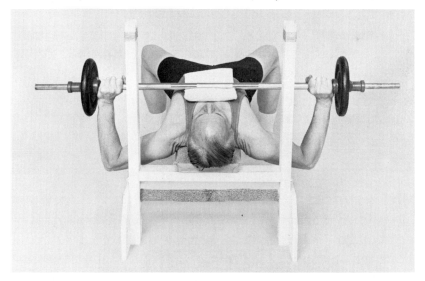

End view, barbell lowered to chest, arms flexed, shows wide hand hold.

Number of Repetitions

To start: 3×, using bar alone or with added weights as indicated above.

Intermediate Level is reached according to the following schedule:

1st 2 weeks 3×
3rd week 4×
4th week 5×
5th week 3×, rest (less than 1 min.), 3×
6th week 4×, rest, 4×
7th week 5×, rest, 5×
8th week 6×, rest, 6×
9th week 7×, rest, 7×
10th week 8×, rest, 8×
11th week 6×, rest, 6×, rest, 6×
12th week 7×, rest, 7×, rest, 7×
13th week 8×, rest, 8×, rest, 8×
14th–17th week add 5 lbs., do 3 sets 8 reps (In these weeks start reducing rest period to 30 seconds or less and in 17th week, with a 10–20 second rest period, this is your Intermediate Level.)

Now, if you started with the bar alone, you should add 5 lbs. every four weeks until it weighs 50 lbs.

However, if you started with more, you may be able to advance upward after 17th week at 5 lbs. every four weeks up to one-half your weight or 90 lbs., whichever is less, as your Advanced Level for this program. In any case, if you have never worked with weights before, it is important to do the first 13 weeks at the same weight to build a base, since the objective here is muscular endurance and fitness, not huge muscles, which are not developed from proper weight training.

NOW REPEAT THE FIRST EXERCISE

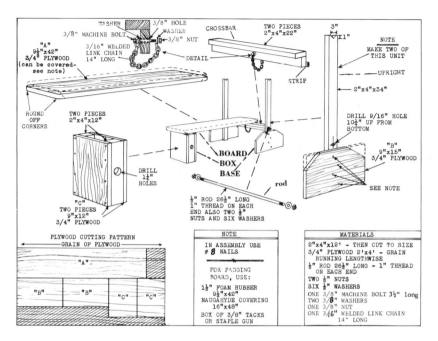

We believe you will find the drawing above and the pictures self-explanatory. We will add a few suggestions:

1. By all means, pad your board. This makes the stand more comfortable.

2. When the barbell is in place in the rack, the bench press has a rather high center of gravity. To counteract this, put one of the dumbbell handles through the chain and attach weights to each end to give the needed stability. As an alternative, any heavy weight can be fastened to the chain for this purpose, provided the bulk of the weight is suspended off the floor.

3. In addition, 1¼-inch holes are drilled in the 2×4s in the box so that a bar can be put through them with weights on each end to give stability if needed.

4. Do not nail the cross bar to the uprights. When you tighten the nuts on the rod, the base becomes one rigid unit. To take apart, just loosen the rod nuts.

THE ALTERNATE
(Advanced Push-ups)

If you do not buy or build a bench press, a program of advanced push-ups can be very effective. However, to start this exercise it should be done exactly as the ninth in the first series, which is as follows:

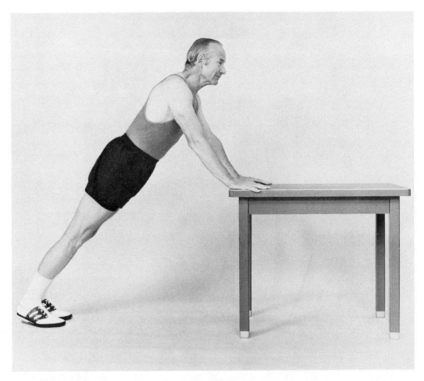

Having made sure your table is strong and won't slide or tip, lean forward with your back straight and place your hands on it.

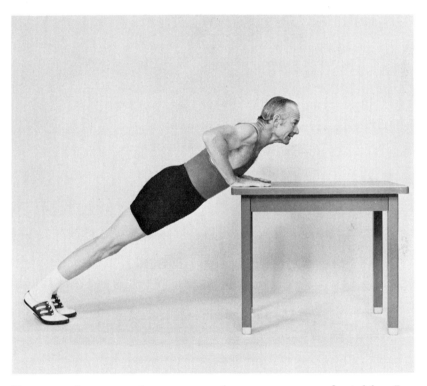

Do a push-up at whatever angle you can comfortably. Inhale going down.

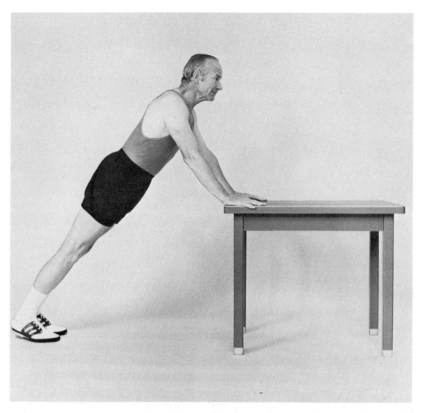

Exhale coming up. Be sure to keep your back straight at all times and look at the wall in front of you, not at the floor. When you can do ten repetitions easily, move your feet away from the table. The ultimate is to do them on the floor touching your chest each time.

Number of Repetitions

To start: 5×
Intermediate Level is reached according to the following schedule:

   By adding one push-up per week for ten weeks you will reach 15, and you should then move to the floor using a 1½ inch wooden block (or two books of the same size).

These push-ups have the advantage, as does the bench press exercise, of stretching the pectoral muscles as far back as possible. The traditional push-up on the floor, particularly if you don't go down all the way, may tend to shorten them. This problem is overcome by using the blocks or books for your hands. Then on each movement go down until your chest touches the floor, looking at the wall ahead. Later, when you approach the advanced level, your feet should go on a block at the same level as the hand blocks or higher, otherwise, you won't get the same effect as with the bench press. In a normal push-up on the floor, the feet take nearly half the weight, so raising them will help to put more of your weight on your hands. So follow this schedule after the tenth week:

11th week, using blocks for hands, look at the wall ahead and touch chest to floor 6×, rest (less than 1 min.), 6×

12th week, 7×, rest, 7×

13th week, 8×, rest, 8× (This is a very strenuous progression, if it is too difficult, take an extra week at each level.)

14th week, 6×, rest, 6×, rest, 6×

15th week, 7×, rest, 7×, rest, 7×

16th week, 8×, rest, 8×, rest, 8×

17th week, 8×, rest, 8×, rest, 8× (In this week start reducing rest periods to 30 seconds or less and when you can do 8×, rest, 8×, rest, 8× with a 10–20 second rest period, this is your Intermediate Level.)

To reach Advanced Level, first put your feet up on a wooden block, then raise them with more blocks or books gradually until you can do 8×, rest, 8×, rest, 8×, with your feet on the chair you use for sit-ups.

NOW REPEAT THE FIRST EXERCISE

INTERMEDIATE AND ADVANCED LEVELS
FOR GFE WITH DUMBBELLS
AND BARBELL

The Intermediate Level is the lowest level at which you can keep sensibly fit, and the Advanced Level is the recommended level for good sound fitness, using as a guide the Time Frame chart on page 118.

INTERMEDIATE LEVEL

No.	Exercise	Number of Reps	Times per Week
1.	Arms Flinging	25	4
2.	Knee Extension and Flexion	12 each side	4
3.	Alternate Knee Raise	12 each side	4
4.	Double Knee Raise	15	4
5.	Hands Overhead, Swinging to the Floor	15 each side	4
6.	Back Exercises (a) through (g)	10 each	4
7.	Figure 8	15 each side	4
8.	Sit-ups	20, hands behind head, no weight	4
9.	Lifts	8×, rest, 8×, rest, 8× (Weight: Bar with sleeve, locking collars and 5 lbs. —2 2½-pound weights)	4
10.	Half-Knee Bends	8×, rest, 8×, rest, 8× (Weight: Bar with sleeve, locking collars and 5 lbs. —2 2½-pound weights)	4

INTERMEDIATE LEVEL (Cont.)

No.	Exercise	Number of Reps	Times per Week
11.	Lift from Floor to Overhead	8×, rest, 8×, rest, 8× (Weight: Bar with sleeve, locking collars and 5 lbs. —2 2½-pound weights)	4
12.	Overhead Press	8×, rest, 8×, rest, 8× (Weight: Bar with sleeve, locking collars and 5 lbs. —2 2½-pound weights)	4
13.	Biceps Curl	8×, rest, 8×, rest, 8× (Weight: Bar with sleeve, locking collars and 5 lbs. —2 2½-pound weights)	4
14.	Bench Press	8×, rest, 8×, rest, 8× (Weight: Bar with sleeve, locking collars and 5 lbs. —2 2½-pound weights)	4
	(or alternate)		
14A.	Advanced Push-ups	Reps as above (Weight: none)	4
	Repeat First Exercise	25—no weight	4

ADVANCED LEVEL

No.	Exercise	Number of Reps.		Times per Week
1.	Arms Flinging	50		3
2.	Knee Extension and Flexion	20	each side	3
3.	Alternate Knee Raise	20	each side	3
4.	Double Knee Raise	20		3
5.	Hands Overhead, Swinging to the Floor	20	each side	3
6.	Back Exercises (a) through (g)	15	each	3
7.	Figure 8	40	each side	3
8.	Sit-ups	40	with 15 lbs. behind head	3
9.	Lifts	8×, rest, 8×, rest, 8× (Weight: one-half your weight or 90 lbs., whichever is less)		3
10.	Half-Knee Bends	8×, rest, 8×, rest, 8× (Weight: one-half your weight or 90 lbs., whichever is less)		3

ADVANCED LEVEL (Cont.)

No.	Exercise	Number of Reps.	Times per Week
11.	Lift from Floor to Overhead	Reps same as above (Weight: one-third your weight)	3
12.	Overhead Press	Reps same as above (Weight: one-third your weight)	3
13.	Biceps Curl	Reps same as above (Weight: one-fourth your weight)	3
14.	Bench Press	Reps same as above (Weight: one-half your weight or 90 lbs., whichever is less)	3
	(or alternate)		
14A.	Advanced Push-ups	Reps same as above (Weight: None but put feet up on chair)	3
	Repeat First Exercise	50—no weight	3

TIME FRAME
(GFE With Dumbbells and Barbell)

Time in Minutes

Week	*Through Age 39*	*Age 40–55*	*Age 56 and up*
1	7	7½	8
2	6½	7	7½
3	7	7½	8
4	7½	8	8½
5	10	10½	11
6	10½	11	11½
7	11	11½	12
8	11½	12	12½
9	12	12½	13
10	12½	13	13½
11	14½	15	15½
12	15	15½	16
13	15½	16	16½
14	17½	18	18½
15	17	17½	18
16	16½	17	17½
17 (Intermediate Level)	16	16½	17
18	18½	19	19½
19	18	18½	19
20	17½	18	18½
21	17	17½	18
22	19½	20	20½
23	19	19½	20
24	18½	19	19½
25*	18	18½	19
42 and up (Advanced Level)	26	27	27½

* Use a steady progression from 25th week up to Advanced Level.

8 | Aerobic or Cardio-pulmonary Exercise (CPE)

WALKING–RUNNING PROGRAM

Of all the exercises in the world, walking and running are the best for all purposes. The use of the legs is basic to achieving aerobic response, and our natural means of loco-motion is the most productive, simplest, and least expensive. The GFE are discussed first because they are done first, but the foundation of a fitness program is the CPE, and walking and running is the cornerstone of that foundation.

When you have finished your general fitness exercises, go for a brisk walk for about 10 minutes according to the chart below. You should cover about six-tenths of a mile, or about 1,000 yards. In winter, keep your cold weather or rain clothes handy because this is an every day part of the program, rain or shine.

Increase the walk one-tenth of a mile per week up to 1½ miles. In the under-30 bracket, this is 4 mph, which is a very quick walk, so time yourself.

TIME IN MINUTES

Week	Distance in Miles	Under Age 30	Age 30–39	Age 40–55	Age 56 and over
1	0.6	9	10½	11	11½
2	0.7	10½	12	12½	13
3	0.8	12	13½	14	14½
4	0.9	13½	15	15½	16
5	1.0	15	16½	17	17½
6	1.1	16½	18	18½	19
7	1.2	18	19½	20	20½
8	1.3	19½	21	21½	22
9	1.4	21	22½	23	23½
10	1.5	22½	24	24½	25

At the beginning of your eleventh week, if you are coming along well with your program and feel fine, you should now start to jog. Pace out 50 yards (25 yards for age 40 and over) so you know what it looks like and jog 50 (or 25) yards and walk 100. (Get someone to drive alongside for a short distance until you get the idea of 4½–5 mph jog. If this is too fast, go as slow as you can and still jog.) *Remember the precautions.* If you feel queer, dizzy, seasick, tightness in your chest, or your heart starts to pound, stop and walk slowly home and check with your doctor.

Shoes

Up to this point you can walk in street shoes, or even a good pair of tennis shoes, but from here on you need a good pair of training shoes in your size and *correct width*. They should have a ¼-inch heel lift, preferably built in. For example, JSF was entered in the Boston Marathon and his shoes were lost in the mail. He went to a local shoe company, which fortunately had his freak size, 11-EEE, and bought a new pair that felt right immediately and which he wore for the first time in the race and went the 26.2 miles without a blister. However, if you have flat feet, you will need jogging shoes that contain a well built-up, soft arch support to prevent arch strain and arch-area blisters. Should foot or knee problems develop, see a podiatrist who normally treats runners' injuries. Most of these arise because the foot is striking the ground at the wrong angle. Such a podiatrist will analyze your feet and give you made-to-order inserts, which should correct this angle and solve your problem.

At this stage of your career you should be able to increase the jog portion about 10 yards a week. This gives you two and a half to three months to get up to jogging 1½ miles. From then on add one-tenth of a mile a week up to 2 miles. You are now at your Intermediate Level distance and should be doing it in about 25–26 minutes.

At about this stage, send for and read an excellent booklet entitled, "Beginning Running." It is booklet number 15 published by *Runner's World* (P.O. Box 366, Mountain View, California 94040). Written by runners with a technically professional approach, it gives a variety of sound concepts about running. This booklet, however, is considerably more sophisticated than its name implies, so, as in this whole program, don't go at it like a tiger.

Your fitness objective is now a shade under 20 minutes for the 2 miles and if you're feeling well you should get there in two more months. At this level, you are doing, on Dr. Kenneth H. Cooper's point system, 2 miles at 9 points × 5 miles a week, for an excellent total of 45 points per week. (One precaution: If you live at an altitude over 4,000 feet, the jogging may bother you. However, if you start very gradually you will acclimatize to it. It will just take longer. On the other hand if you go visiting in a place at any altitude, reduce your distance drastically and go very slowly for a few days until you get used to it.)

During this period you may feel a little tired from time to time. The schedule can come down to 5 × a week, but in no case below 4 ×. To vary the program and to speed recovery, try doing the GFE on the off days.

When you are running your 40 points a week, you are statistically fit in terms of the general U.S. population, if not in terms of competition. Furthermore, by now you should know yourself and your limitations. If you are just not feeling right, it is plain good sense to stop during a workout. Besides the obvious one, another good reason to stop when you are uncertain is that if you love the sport you don't want to hurt it by becoming a nonvital statistic. Properly checked by your doctor, at least annually, you can add a mile or so a month to each run. Add mileage like this for six months, if 25–35 years old; over 35, add a mile every other month, using your judgment about not getting over-tired. Run long and slow during this time, reading these books in the order listed:

The Stress of Life, Hans Selye, M.D. (New York: McGraw-Hill, 1956).

"Athlete and Adaptation to Stress," Forbes Carlile, from *Run, Run, Run,* by Fred Wilt (Los Altos, California: Track and Field News, 1964).

Aerobics, Kenneth H. Cooper, M.D., M.P.H. (New York: M. Evans, 1968).

The Conditioning of Distance Runners, Thomas J. Osler (A Long Distance Log Publication, 1967, United States Track and Field Federation, P.O. Box 190, Tucson, Arizona 85702).

Strength, Power and Muscular Endurance for Runners and Hurdlers, John P. Jesse (San Marino, California: Athletic Press, [a Division of Golden West Books], 1971). Only 157 pages, this is a highly advanced and thoroughly sophisticated book on calisthenics and weight training, specifically for runners. Note, especially, exercises 31 and 32 on page 114, which strengthen both the quadriceps group on the front of the thigh and the hamstring group on the back. Generally, the preponderance of runners will have stronger hamstrings than quadriceps and should emphasize the extensions, doing more reps and working up to heavier weights. On the other hand, those who have stronger quadriceps should do just the reverse. This is known as keeping the antagonists in balance. There is one precaution, however. Start with light weight and increase it very gradually to avoid strain and injury.

The above are the main courses for the information-hungry jogger, and here are some delightful in-between snacks:

Long Slow Distance: The Humane Way to Train, Joe Henderson (Los Altos, California: Tafnews Press, 1970).

Road Racers and Their Training, edited by Joe Henderson (Los Altos, California: Tafnews Press, 1970).

Four Million Footsteps, Bruce Tulloh (London: Mayflower Books, 1970).

On the Run from Dogs and People, Hal Higdon (Chicago: Henry Regnery Company, 1971).

Runner's World (magazine), P.O. Box 366, Mountain View, Calif. 94040.

Guide to Distance Running, edited by Joe Henderson and Bob Anderson (Mountain View, Calif.: *Runner's World* Magazine, 1971).

Learn from Dr. Selye how your body reacts with resistance to the stressor, which in this case is running, under the general adaptation syndrome, and learn to stop short of exhaustion. Learn how Dr. Cooper shook the athletic world with his concept of cardiopulmonary fitness and the training effect. Then see how Carlile and Osler carry these into a practical program. If you get this far, you will start to vary your daily mileage and will develop your own program.

The books by these authors will explain why running has been stressed here as the best aerobic exercise—because it is the most practical and the least expensive. If it is absolutely impossible to find a place to run (living on the twentieth floor of an apartment house in a congested area), there are two choices: run in place or get a treadmill.

Running in place has the advantage of convenience, but there are some precautions that must be taken. You should have a soft rug with a rubber mat to run on and shoes with a sponge-rubber sole. The count is taken when the left foot hits the ground and the feet must clear the ground by 8 inches. This is a very high step and it is difficult to keep up for the long periods necessary in this exercise. It can also be hard on the ankles and feet, particularly for older people. If this is your only solution, I suggest you get a copy of Dr. Cooper's *New Aerobics* and follow the detailed schedule in his "Chart Pack."

A motor-driven treadmill costs from $400–$1,600, and the type that will permit you to reach the 6 mph speed for 2 miles in 20 minutes start at around $525. This is an excellent solution if you wish to make the investment. It will have a recording device so you can use it according to the regular program. Since running on a treadmill isn't too exciting, set it up in front of the television or where you can hear your radio or stereo.

BIKE PROGRAM
Out-of-Doors

The theory that you don't forget how to ride a bike is reasonably true, but if you haven't done it consistently your muscles will have softened up. "We rode bikes when we went to Bermuda in 1968" won't do it either. So start off gently. Don't buy a bike until you are sure this is your definite selection for CPE. Borrow or rent one, because the rate of disuse of exercising equipment is pretty high and an expensive bike in the cellar or attic ties up a lot of money. In any case, measure out 2 miles in your car and figure it so you can add miles with reasonable accuracy. Start out with 2 miles in 12 minutes or slightly under and hold this level for three weeks. If you feel well, add ¼ mile a week for four weeks; then start to pick up speed gradually until you can do 5-minute miles or $3 \times 5 = 15$ minutes. Then add distance: half a mile a week. Your time will go up and, when it does, hold that distance until your time is down to 5 minutes per mile. This will be harder as you increase but your objective is to reach 10 miles in 50 minutes or less, giving 5 points per day × 6 times a week for a very good total of 30 points on Dr. Cooper's point system. Bike riding inevitably will take more time than running or swimming. Even so, it is a great sport, if the trails or paths are available.

Indoors

If there are no paths or bike trails in your area and it is still your selection, you will need a stationary bicycle with a timer, speedometer, and mileage indicator. Current prices range from about $100 on up. However, there is no need at the outset to get an extremely expensive one. There is a very good one (Schwinn Deluxe Exerciser, Model XR-5) with speedometer, mileage indicator, timer, and adjustable resistance control. It costs $128.95 plus state and local taxes, and will be fine for your purposes. Whatever you do, get one with stationary handlebars. On some types the handlebars go up and down, presumably to give more exercise. As a result, the resistance on one foot is nearly twice what it is on the other, creating an unacceptable imbalance. In any case, set your stationary bike up in front of the TV or near the radio or stereo, so you will be entertained while you are "riding"; work out your speed and distance schedule and pedal away.

SWIMMING PROGRAM

If this sport is your choice, it is assumed you know how to swim and that you enjoy it, otherwise you would hardly select swimming as your CPE; also that there is an indoor pool available, or you live near other all-year swimming facilities.

The following program is based on the overhand crawl:

Measure the pool so that you know how many laps represent 100 yards, 200 yards, etc. Start out by swimming 100 yards in 3 minutes or less. Do this for two weeks. Gradually increase your speed and reduce your time so you can do it in 2½ minutes; then add 25 yards a week until you get up to 200 yards. Your time per 100 yards will tend to increase, so try to keep it down to 2½ minutes per 100 yards. When you can do the 200 yards in 5 minutes, then start adding 25 yards a week, trying to maintain the speed. The objective is to reach 800 yards and be able to do it slightly under 20 minutes for 6½ Cooper points; 5× a week gives you 32½ points which, with your GFE, will keep you in splendid shape.

Swimming is excellent if you are lucky enough to have a pool available. Just follow the program and use it as your aerobic exercise. Many prefer it because of its overall use of the muscles.

GENERAL CONSIDERATIONS
Posture

Raise your chest up in a manner that was demonstrated by an instructor, who used to come over and grab a few hairs on a young man's chest and pull up at a 45° angle. When the trainee reached the correct position, the pull was relaxed, to his considerable relief.

Flatten your seat by pushing it forward so the back is

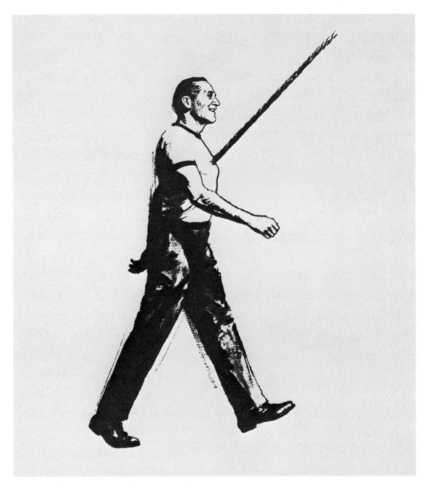

Excellent walking posture.

flat and not arched, and as part of this position the upper
and lower abdomen are drawn up and in.

Raising the chest is fairly easy after some practice and
self-reminders, but flattening the seat takes a lot of work
and may not be reached until the abdominal muscles are fit.

Proper posture should be practiced along with the exercises for two reasons: for appearance; and to take the strain and pressure off your back by balancing your weight evenly. Otherwise, you arch your back into a strained position. This is exactly what happens when someone carries an excess tummy out in front.

Time of Day

The best time to exercise is early morning after the calls of nature. Then, after the workout, you have a few minutes to simmer down while bathing and shaving or, in the case of women, making up.

When you come home from work is also a good time for your workout because it unwinds the tensions of the day. However, when daylight saving time ends, winter darkness can pose a problem. However, there are parks and school tracks and gyms, although outdoors is preferable.

Colds or Minor Illnesses

In the first period of a cold (not requiring a doctor's visit), when you are sneezing or pouring from the head, all exercise should be skipped. Your body is under sufficient general stress from the cold. However, once your cold has loosened up and you begin to feel well again, the best advice We've heard is given by Thomas J. Osler in his excellent little book *The Conditioning of Distance Runners*. Take the number of days you missed exercise and divide it into the number of exercises (or the distance you have been running) and that is your first day's workout. Example: You have been out four days. You have been doing 15 of an exercise; do four to start. You have been walking or running 1 mile; go one-quarter to start. The next day, if you feel even better, add another one-quarter, and the same each day until you are back on schedule. However, if you don't feel right, lay off another day or two until you get your pep back. Be most careful exercising after a cough. The inflammation is in a danger area and it should be cleared up before you start again.

A word of caution is needed about your "friends" and colds. You may get this gratuitous comment: "I thought you would be in such good shape you'd never get a cold." This is a needling remark that is telling you your program is useless and you're wasting your time, so ignore it. No one understands the cold. For most people, being in good shape lessens the chance of getting a cold, provided one doesn't get too tired, and it also lessens the duration and the intensity of the cold. Get exhausted and you'll catch a cold sooner or later. Short exposures to cold in the early fall help build resistance, but this is tricky. You have to know your limits very well so as not to overdo it.

Clothes

If your CPE program is walking–running or bicycling, don't buy a lot of special clothes right away. Use your old ones. In summer that old worn knit sports shirt you were going to throw away and some shorts will do. Use regular underwear to prevent chafing. If you don't have a pair of shorts, cut off a pair of old slacks about 4–6 inches above the top of the knee cap. A 3-inch vent in the side seam will give freer movement of the legs. If you're not happy about the appearance of your legs, don't cut the slacks off for a while.

Above all, clothes should be loose and easy to permit free movement. In winter, an old wool sweater (as much real wool as possible), with a soft undershirt and a loose pair of slacks, will do until it gets very cold. When it gets much below 20°F. you should wear some wool or "thermal" underwear, ankle length, for plenty of protection. Men must make sure the groin is well covered in very cold weather. Some men can run in a supporter. Others can't. Women can wear wool panties under a loose pair of slacks. Most women runners say it's more comfortable to wear a bra under the sweater and a little undershirt, according to the weather. (Whatever you wear and regardless of the season, inner clothing that touches the skin should be washed out after every workout. It will pay dividends by avoiding the myriad of low-grade fungus infections that thrive in damp, dirty athletic clothes.)

Actually, when you get used to it, you can walk and run in shorts until fairly late in the season; if there is no wind, down to about 35°F. Mineral oil on the legs helps, but this is a lot of bother.

SALINE (ELECTROLYTE) AND FLUID MANAGEMENT*

Even with the modest programs suggested in this chapter, it is a good idea to have some knowledge of this subject, especially for hot weather. The great professional runner, Bill Emmerton, has run through Death Valley, which proves what the ultimate in fitness can accomplish for its proud possessor, but not being that fit we must exercise with precaution in hot weather.

* For a more detailed discussion of this subject, see Chapter 11.

Before any strenuous exercise in hot, or even warm weather, take three 8-ounce glasses of cool (not cold) water over a half-hour period with two dissolved or completely chewed-up 500 mg. (7½ grains) salt tablets. During the activity, take two glasses every 30–45 minutes (depending on strenuousness of the exercises) with one more salt tablet, again dissolved or chewed up. After exercise, keep drinking lots more water. If exertion was very prolonged (3 or 4 hours) you may need some more salt, but as you get more fit you can and should definitely cut the amount of salt in half; never the water. It is a good idea to weigh yourself before and after workouts, to get an idea of how much water you lose. You can then replace the fluid (two 8-ounce glasses equal a pound). Your scales are your best guide to the volume of fluid replacement.

COOLING OFF AFTER EXERCISE

After a good workout and a run, your body needs a few minutes to readjust. Don't under any circumstances, jump into a car immediately and drive off, or get into a tub or shower. Instead do the following:

If you have time, walk a couple of hundred yards at a modest pace. If time is short, go inside, get on the floor and raising your legs and rear end off the floor, prop yourself up with your hands to get your legs as high as possible; bicycle smoothly 100 times, rest a minute, and do another 100. Bring your feet down and sit up a few seconds. Then stand up slowly. The reason for this is that during the run 50–70 percent of the blood in your body is in your legs. It is pumped down by the heart and squeezed back by the contraction of muscles in the legs. When you stop, your heart is still pumping fairly hard, but there are no muscle contractions to help push the blood back, so it pools in the legs. We have often heard of soldiers fainting in formation. This is the result of blood pooling in the legs and insufficient blood in the brain. The same thing can happen after a hard run. The walk and the bicycle exercise recirculate and redistribute the blood so this doesn't happen.

EATING

Never exercise right after a meal. The amount of time to wait depends largely on the size of the meal. If one alcoholic drink of any kind has been consumed, wait until the next day.

As far as food is concerned:

After a small sandwich and a glass of skim milk, wait 1½ hours;

After a light meal of food you can digest easily, wait 2½ hours;

After an old-fashioned Thanksgiving Dinner, wait 4 hours, or exercise beforehand. (Many people make a rule of waiting 4 hours even after an average meal.)

SOME ADVICE TO THE OLDER EXERCISER

A few years ago, a tough old professional athlete was giving instructions in weight training to a paunchy businessman, who was complaining that he was "too old for that sort of thing."

Without a word, the pro showed him a photograph of a

white-haired man of eighty on a bench press, pressing his age plus a hundred pounds.

The businessman asked, "How can a man of that age do it?"

Giving him a hard look, the pro answered, "Age has got nothing to do with it."

The man knew the pro to be an expert in physical education, who understood the cellular aging process as well as anyone. What he had heard was a tough piece of philosophy, an attitude toward life, which we should all try to adopt.

"Age has got nothing to do with it." Don't worry about it; don't think about it, and above all, don't talk about it, especially to younger people. Most of them will automatically give you the respect you think you deserve for the difference in age, but they will respect you a lot more if you never mention it.

The man who says: "Why I did so and so before you were born," or, "When I was your age," etc., is nothing but a crashing bore. If a man has to boast about his age, he probably hasn't much else to be proud of.

Associate when you can with younger people; try to see their point of view and even be able to talk their language so you have communication and understanding, and at the same time keep the balance and maturity that the few extra years should have given you. When you get in really good shape, you might exercise with a younger man who is just starting. Your superior fitness will give him a challenge, and whether he excels you or not isn't important as long as you have companions and eventually a few younger friends.

Excess fatigue can sometimes creep into an exercise program from being physically or mentally tired, or any combination of both. If you feel logy and disspirited and the program is twice as hard to go through, figure out a completely new route for the run. If this doesn't help, take two days off in a row and do something with your wife, husband, or friend that is totally different and, if possible, intellectually stimulating. See a good show, go to a concert if you like music, attend a lecture on your favorite subject, see an art exhibition—something that is fun. Enjoy life, but don't overdo or take it as an excuse to stay up all night and celebrate. The idea is to get rested and refreshed, not more exhausted. Then go back and resume your program. Normally, a respite of two days should cure the problem, provided you get enough sleep at night. But if it hasn't, try taking a short nap, or lie down when you get home in the evening or during the day over weekends. The additional rest should help you adapt to the stress of the exercise as well as to the other stresses of your life and reach a healthy balance between rest and work. But, above all, don't let anyone tell you to lay off for a month or two to "take a rest," because that isn't a rest—that's quitting. To keep up enthusiasm, find out who else in the neighborhood has a program. Get to know them and talk to them. Read the literature of your sport and of fitness in general. The group association is the best because it provides companionship, good-natured competition, and stimulates enthusiasm.

9 | The Nutrition

The next time you see your doctor, ask him about diet. He will tell you of any restrictions due to your physical condition and will give you general guidelines on how much to eat. Using those guidelines, this chapter will give you a balanced-diet approach to planning meals.

If you are overweight, with fat that is, the one basic rule you must follow is to cut down, not out. This does not mean that you shouldn't eliminate refined sugars and foods from your diet, because they are incomplete foods from which much important nutrition has been cut out. From a nutritional standpoint, the "cut-out" diets vary from unsound to fraudulent and dangerous. Some of them work initially because you are motivated and tend to hold back on intake, but the great danger of these high protein and low fat carbohydrate diets is that they upset normal metabolism with increased production of ketones, which suppresses appetite.

With his appetite very much reduced, the dieter loses weight and is delighted with the results. The only problem is that he now has a metabolic pattern similar to diabetes. One such dieter blacked out when getting out of the bathtub, fell, hit his head, and was nearly drowned.

A well-known diet of this type, which is in *Dr. Atkins Diet Revolution . . .* , has been condemned by the Council of Foods and Nutrition, of the American Medical Association, as being without merit and fraught with hazards. Despite the siren song of the purveyors of these fast-buck diet books, it is far safer and better to get motivated on a sound basis. Then you will improve your health, enjoy eating, and get that marvelous sense of well-being that comes with good diet plus exercise.

The amount you eat should be related to your energy output as well as your size and present weight. Cadets at West Point can eat 4,000 to 4,500 calories a day and be as hard as rocks; so can Finnish lumberjacks and Swiss Alpine mountaineers. But a completely inactive sedentary person is in a tough position. It is almost impossible for him to cut down enough to balance his calorie intake with his physical output and still get sufficient nutrients and vitamins to remain healthy. If he weighs 150 pounds, and can eat only 1,800 calories per day if he wants to stay even, he will be limiting his selection of foods as well as his intake.

On the other hand, if he becomes normally active and conscientiously walks as much during the day as time will permit and does ample regular exercise on a planned basis, he can eat several hundred extra calories a day and still stay even. With this extra margin, he should regularly have a wider spectrum of foods and, on a rare occasion, doesn't need to offend his hostess by turning down the flaming cherries jubilee or ice cream. He can eat four slices of whole grain bread without a qualm and have a diet with every kind of nutrition, vitamins and minerals. But without this extra activity, his circulatory system, organs, and musculoskeletal system are going to suffer from the lack of movement and the lack of circulation. So he is in an unpromising situation and headed for trouble unless he alters his way of living.

The Magic Numbers

Your calorie balance, like your fingerprints, is different from everyone else's. But, unlike your fingerprints, there are some standards that apply to most people that you need to know to find your magic number and set a proper intake level. Each person burns a certain amount of fuel to keep his motors idling (basal metabolism). On top of that fuel consumption, there are power demands for extra fuel for every form of physical activity: household, shopping, walking, office, sales, and sports and exercise, and there are charts to measure various activities. (See Appendix, *Amount of Calories Expended.*) To determine your magic number, take your weight stripped, after the bathroom but before breakfast. If you are a moderately active person, a busy housewife with two or three kids who does it all herself, or the husband who walks as much as possible between appointments and gets in some modest outdoor activity in the evenings and on weekends (short of a regular program of exercise), you can multiply your weight by 15. If a man weighs 180 pounds, 180 times 15 equals 2,700. For a less active woman, multiply by 13. At age 30, this number of total calories (including those drinks) will keep you even. In *Overweight Causes, Cost, and Control,* Dr. Jean Mayer suggests that older people, assuming less maintenance fuel and less activity, should deduct some percentage of calories for every ten years over age 25.

However, the rule of 15 is only a starter. Use the tables and see what you have been eating. If you weigh 160 pounds and have been maintaining your weight at 2,400 calories a day, the rule works perfectly. If you have been gaining at 2,400, try 13 × 160 and create a calorie deficit from that level; but no more reduction than 250–500 calories per day. Because of danger to health and poor results, including our own experience, we are against high-calorie deficits. Some years ago JSF went for a medical checkup after a long period of neglect. Blood pressure was up, cholesterol was over 300, and, at 210 pounds, he was about 30 pounds too heavy. He had been exercising sporadically with weights, but not enough to offset a high-calorie intake. With strict orders to lose, he tried an 1,800-calorie diet; 210 × 15 = 3,150, which should have been his balance point. With a deficit of about 1,350 calories a day, he should have lost 2½ to 3 pounds a week, but keeping to that level was so difficult he nearly gave up. Finally, he settled on 2,500–2,600 calories a day, stepped up his exercise with a three-times-a-week jogging program and was down to 190 in three months. Then in his early fifties, he felt better than when he was 25, and the program really took hold. As his exercise increased, he found he could hold his weight or even lose a little on 3,000 calories a day. A number of years later, when his jogging and running lengthened to about 60 miles a week, he kept in balance on 4,000 calories a day.

The point here is that the body has in it a regulatory

system called homeostasis (the tendency of the body to maintain things as they are), which operates independently of a consciously planned diet program. In times of severe hunger, the body can adjust, burn less, and get along on extremely low-calorie levels, as prisoners of war found out. On the other hand, with an excessive diet, the body will both burn more and store fat as if against a possible period of low nutrition. Furthermore, a sedentary person on a 2,000-calorie diet with a 250-calorie daily deficit will store more and burn less than a strenuous exerciser on a 3,000-calorie diet with the same 250-calorie deficit.

These adaptive mechanisms tend to alter the straight calorie consumption and the calorie-deficit ratios, which is the reason so many people get discouraged early in a diet and exercise program when "nothing happens." It is as if the body were saying, "I'm from Missouri; I'm going to wait and make you prove that you really mean it." Then, when the body finally decides you do, after staying at a level from which it has refused to move, you may get a sudden and very encouraging drop. Farther along in the program, mentally charged up by his progress, the dieter gets a feel for how much to eat and settles into a routine on which it is really very easy to keep weight in balance, especially when on a good exercise program. There is a regulatory system in the brain operated by a satiety center, which controls appetite and signals that feeling of fullness.

As an example of how this works, after a prolonged, strenuous exercise session, you should wait at least half an hour before eating. Then you'll be hungry and can eat a 1,000-calorie meal without any discomfort. On a day when you haven't exercised, at around 500–700 calories you'll probably start to feel stuffed and if you don't stop eating you'll become very uncomfortable. The satiety mechanism works very accurately when you are on a heavy exercise schedule.

If the dieter who has been maintaining level weight reduces his intake by 250 calories a day, he'll lose about half a pound a week. Unless the doctor has advised more, this isn't a bad objective because weight lost slowly is more apt to stay off for many reasons. It would probably do no harm to reduce 500 calories per day and lose a pound a week. But remember that this program is lifetime, to be lived with and enjoyed; so try to keep it in that bracket. Crash diets, unless under direct medical supervision, are vicious, dangerous, and futile because the weight nearly always goes back on and, when it does, this "rhythm method of girth control" just raises Cain with your cardiovascular system, blood lipids (blood fat), and the whole works. Just don't do it!

The Composition of Foods

Within the framework of these general rules, you can go into calorie counting to your heart's content. Rather than print a detailed chart of calories here, we recommend that you write to the Superintendent of Documents, U.S. Government Printing Office, Washington, D.C. 20402 and ask for *Composition of Foods—Raw, Processed, Prepared,* Agriculture Handbook No. 8, Agricultural Research Service, United States Department of Agriculture. The cost of the handbook at this writing is only $3.60. You can pay many times that in a store for books on diets and you won't get as accurate or as detailed a picture of the calories in, or composition of, almost every food you can think of.

One of the basic rules of diet is to eat three meals a day. You often hear the chorus, especially from women,

"Oh, I can't eat breakfast; just can't face it." Or from the men, "I skip lunch because I'm on the run; I save calories that way." They are both wrong. The women should coax themselves out of the nonbreakfast habit with small delicious things, which may be a compromise with the calorie total until the breakfast habit is firmly established. Dr. Benjamin F. Miller in his *Complete Medical Guide* has one of the most sensible approaches to this problem, which is starting 15 minutes earlier in the morning and making breakfast a really tasty and enjoyable experience. As for the man "on the run," he is going to save time if he stops for a light lunch. Not only will he avoid that inevitable afternoon letdown, which results from low blood sugar, but the improvement in his efficiency will more than make up for the minutes spent at lunch.

Why three meals? The reasons are basic. You were probably brought up that way and your system is used to the spacing and timing of meals and sleep. Furthermore, with irregular or skipped meals the body will store, as fat, more of the calories consumed. For example, if a man eats 2,500 calories, evenly spaced through the day, his body will store less fat than if he ate a 500-calorie breakfast, skipped lunch, and gorged himself with a 2,000-calorie evening meal, given the same amount of activity in both cases. This was demonstrated first by Dr. Clarence Cohn on rats, and then with people by Dr. E. S. Gordon. The reasons for this are obscure, but in times of famine the body may have learned to store some portion of what food it did get as a reserve against foodless days. Consequently, with skipped meals it may signal an emergency that sends food to the storehouse. Another reason for eating regularly is shown by what happens when you fly across the country or abroad and change all your meal and sleep times around.

Unless you allow adequate rest, eat sensibly, and adjust gradually to the time change, you'll be a basket case for a few days, as so many aggressive American businessmen have found out.

The next rule of diet is to eat slowly and chew your food properly. This does several things. In order to eat slowly, you have to throttle down all those revved-up motors. The extra time taken eating slowly will be saved after the meal because you won't be fussing over indigestion. Furthermore, it gives that little satiety gland that controls your appetite time to get working. You'll be satisfied with less food and your body will get more nourishment from it. Some of the nonsense you have to listen to on this subject includes: "I learned to eat fast in the 'Service.'" "I don't fool around when I eat; my time is money." These remarks are boasting and self-indicting.

When you embark on a regular program of exercise, you may find that you can adjust calorie balance by meeting the rule of 15, or by being, say, 100 calories a day under it until you reach your desired weight. If your program is quite vigorous, the desired weight may be on the upper side of the weight chart, because muscle weighs nearly one and a half times as much as fat, and bones tend to weigh more as they toughen up with added calcium due to exercise. Adjustment in your intake can be handled by a little judicious use of *Composition of Foods* mentioned above.

One old wives' tale often comes from the friend who hears you are on a diet and offers: "You'll have to shrink your stomach, you know." Just tell him his head is for shrinking but not your stomach; your stomach does fine by itself. Anyway, it's your point of view, not your stomach.

Another old wives' tale is that exercise will give you an uncontrollable appetite. This excuse, like many other excuses for not exercising, is a myth in which the wish is father to the thought. In the first few weeks you may experience a mild increase in appetite, but as you stay on the program the increase in appetite will totally disappear and your appetite, if anything, will diminish below its previous level. This does not mean that your consumption of food will necessarily be the same, as the body will tend to compensate for the increased activity. Since this is a normal adaptive response, your weight eventually stabilizes under the program at a level appropriate to your age, size, and activity. There will be more on this in Chapter 10.

The Seven Food Groups

These groups of food, seven in all, have been expanded from the four food groups that were used for so many years. They have been adapted to conform with developments in the field of nutrition in the last ten years, especially in respect to three important concepts:

1. The widest possible selection of foods is basic to sound nutrition, subject to certain restrictions, which will be brought out below.

2. The seven food groups lead directly away from heavily processed and refined foods, which are both less nutritious and more expensive. In addition, the above developments strongly indicate that it is the lack of certain elements in the diet, rather than the presence of others, which may aid the formation of dangerous fatty deposits in artery walls (atherosclerosis). This underscores the need for a wide selection of foods, and especially to increase dietary fiber.

3. Since excess calories from any source will cause obesity and very often concomitant atherosclerosis, it is

advisable to reduce total fat intake in the diet as one of the means of reducing total caloric consumption and bringing it in line with energy output.

Several methods of minimizing the percentage of fat in the diet are discussed in the ensuing pages. If followed, they will, coincidentally, lower your intake of saturated fat. With this, most doctors will agree. However, if you have been advised by your doctor to substitute some of this saturated fat with cold-pressed, unrefined, polyunsaturated fats, we are not going to argue with him. (The prevalence of processing that involves heat treatment, bleaching, neutralization, or deodorization is so universal that it is extremely difficult to avoid. Thus, unless the consumer buys vegetable oils that specifically state "unrefined cold-pressed," he may be buying and consuming fats that have become saturated and, in fact, will be defeating any objective he may have of avoiding such fats.)

In limited quantities, this substitution seems to be healthful and harmless. On the other hand, there are a few significant people in the medical and scientific fraternity who now believe that the development of atherosclerosis is caused by factors other than a high intake of saturated fats, a theory that certainly seems to be supported by the Blattendorf study mentioned in Chapter 2 (see page 15). These doctors and scientists emphasize the need to avoid obesity, smoking, excessive alcohol, external and internal environmental conditions that lead to high blood pressure, and to exercise sensibly, which are the things this book is all about.

Protein

Most of the world's population is short of the vitally important nutrient, protein, and will be for years to come. They must survive on protein from grains and vegetables, which is known collectively as "vegetable protein."

The United States and a few other wealthy nations get theirs from animal sources. But we cannot count indefinitely on the availability of this costly form of protein. Furthermore, our excessive consumption of it and the fat that goes with it has made us victims of certain illnesses called the diseases of affluence. Consequently, for reasons of health as well as eventual supply, we must begin to think in terms of getting more of our protein from fish and vegetable sources and of relying on animal protein to a decreasing extent.

The selections and combinations of foods in the following pages have been made for optimal nutritional health, with emphasis on the shift to more vegetable protein. You should feel better with it and get better reports from your doctor.

In making this switch in dietary management, it is essential to understand the variability of the biologic value of protein. The amino acids of protein are the building blocks of our body, and like the foundation of a house, things don't work too well if some important blocks are missing.

Some balancing or mutual supplementation of these blocks has occurred in the past for cultural reasons. Those considerations no longer apply in our heterogeneous society, nor are they very accurate. However, we can now balance protein on the basis of the latest scientific information.

Vegetable proteins are generally low in the essential amino acids known as: lysine, tryptophane, methionine, threonine, and occasionally valine. As a result, they will not support normal growth or supply adequate vigor if eaten separately. These vegetable sources are said to have a low biologic value, or net protein utilization (NPU). Fortunately, not all of them are low in all of these aminos, so we can arrange them in combinations that balance. When this is done correctly, the combined total is worth more than the sum of the parts separately. (The Institute of Nutrition of Central America and Panama has developed a well-balanced plant protein mixture called "Incaparina," which has been successfully used in the treatment of kwashiorkor, a protein deficiency disease. It contains 27.5 percent protein, principally from whole ground corn, sorghum, and cottonseed flour, but we doubt if you can find it in the market.)

More specifically, NPU is the percentage of protein that is absorbed by the digestive tract and actually used by the body. Animal protein has an NPU of approximately 75 percent and the vegetable protein about 50 percent, but with the right combinations they will be higher. For a comprehensive explanation of how to achieve optimum combinations, see Frances Moore Lappé's, *Diet for a Small Planet*.

There are many conflicting opinions on how much protein per day is sufficient, and, indeed, this is a badly neglected aspect of the problem. The National Research Council advises 56 grams of protein for an adult male weighing 154 lbs. and 46 grams for a woman weighing 128 lbs. This is equal to an allowance of .8 gram of protein per kilogram of body weight for healthy adults in a temperate climate. However, it doesn't take into account either the quality of the protein or variations in individual biologic needs. The latter can be determined only by a complicated blood and hair analysis, which is a new scientific process.

In the following pages, we have allowed a total of 2,100 calories and an NPU of 62 grams of protein per day, based on an individual of 140 lbs. (see table below). Since the NPU has been figured on the sum of the parts separately, the combined total will be somewhat higher. This should provide a well-balanced mixture of protein for healthy life processes and plenty of vigor with an adequate margin of safety.

Here is a table to determine proportionate amounts of either calories or grams of protein for people of various weights. The indicated portions in each food group equal 100 percent and are for the 140-lb. person:

100 lbs.— 72%	150 lbs.—107%
105 lbs.— 75%	155 lbs.—111%
110 lbs.— 79%	160 lbs.—114%
115 lbs.— 82%	165 lbs.—118%
120 lbs.— 86%	170 lbs.—121%
125 lbs.— 89%	175 lbs.—125%
130 lbs.— 93%	180 lbs.—128%
135 lbs.— 97%	185 lbs.—132%
140 lbs.— 100%	190 lbs.—136%
145 lbs.— 105%	195 lbs.—139%
	200 lbs.—143%

GROUP 1—
WHOLE GRAINS AND CEREALS

"God also said, 'I give you all
plants that bear seed everywhere
on earth, and every tree bearing
fruit which yields seed: they shall
be yours for food.' "

Genesis 1:29

DAILY ALLOWANCE

BREADS (Whole grain only, 2 percent nonfat dry milk added)	Average Calories for Amounts Shown	Average Grams of Protein for Amounts Shown	
4 slices per day, based on a person of 140 lbs.		*Gross Protein*	*NPU*
Whole wheat Whole rye Oatmeal Corn Other whole grain breads Multiple grain breads	275	11.0	5.0
CEREALS (Unrefined) *Cooked* (1 cup per day cooked, with ½ cup skim milk and 2 level tablespoons raw wheat germ) Oatmeal (not the quick cooking kind) Cream of rye (whole) Cornmeal (whole, not degermed) Rice, brown, unpolished	250	12.0	8.0
Uncooked (½ cup per day) Bran mixture	110	10.8	5.8

Bran mixture: One serving, or ¼ cup, consists of 2 level tablespoons of crude bran, 1 of raw wheat germ, and 1 of brewer's yeast. Adding bran to the diet is highly recommended as a result of recent medical and scientific studies, which demonstrate lack of fiber in our diet due to refinement. Fiber is essential for proper elimination and aids in prevention of a number of diseases, now endemic in western society. The bran, wheat germ, and brewer's yeast provide a balanced protein and are excellent sources of vitamins and minerals. To enhance their flavor, mix in some chopped fruit.

In considering this important group, it is essential to understand something about its background, what has happened to it over the years and why. Then you will begin to realize how you have been taken in by the con game being played on you by the milling industry.

The history of grinding wheat and other grains to make flour goes back six thousand years to the early days of the Egyptians. From primitively crushing the grains by hand between two rocks, a less wasteful method evolved of using a mortar and pestle. Much later, in the fourth century B.C., the Greeks and the Romans developed the system of using an upper and nether millstone, operated either by animal or water power.

The product of these ancient mills was always a rough, coarse, whole grain flour, principally of wheat but occasionally of corn. The grain was taken to the mill by the farmer to be ground, where he paid the miller for his services in cash or in a percentage of the flour. These crude mills were used for hundreds of years and were known as grist mills.

In the early nineteenth century the roller mill was invented and about the same time an Austrian named Ignes

Paur designed a machine known as a "middlings purifier," which is what started all the trouble. It separated the outer layers of bran on the wheat kernel, which were then referred to as "highly indigestible." On the contrary, we know today that bran is anything but that. A major percentage of these bran layers consists of highly digestible nutrients, including vitamins, minerals, and a useful protein. Although the cellulose or crude fiber in the bran (9–10 percent) does not digest, it provides necessary bulk in the diet, which aids digestion and elimination by performing an essential mechanical function.

During this period other machines were invented which milled out the germ because the oil in it was thought to turn bread rancid. This is a fallacy, as good quality whole wheat bread, or any bread for that matter, can be stored as long as need be under refrigeration in a tightly closed cellophane bag. This is not to say that long storage of any food is encouraged, because there is almost always a loss of nutritional value in proportion to the length of time in storage.

These facts about wheat flour and bread made from it were not generally known in the last century. Millers persisted in separating out the bran and the germ, calling them "offal" and "impurities," leaving the sterile white flour that is still the bane of our existence today.

One bright spot appeared in this nutritional travesty when a reformer from Connecticut, Sylvester Graham, urged an improvement in the making of bread by using only "unbolted" or whole wheat flour. Graham flour became the name of whole wheat flour and is still used today for flour and for graham crackers, although some millers have taken the name and applied it to an adulterated product made of poor quality flour and bran.

Much of the motive for the early use of white bread came from the misconception that it was more digestible. This was only true in the sense that whole wheat flour contained the coarse vegetable fiber that didn't digest, because nature hadn't put it there for that purpose. It was in the wheat kernel as bulk to help push the mass of partially digested food through the intestines. Even more important, the germ and the bran, which were being processed out, contain large amounts of protein, vitamins, and minerals.

The basic need for these parts of the grain to remain in the diet is recognized by such distinguished scientists and medical men as Roger J. Williams, Ph.D., D.Sc., and Denis P. Burkitt, M.D. Furthermore, a most important event occurred recently when Dr. Jean Mayer went on national television and told the American public to avoid the consumption of refined carbohydrates and to eat, instead, whole grain breads and cereals. These men not only state that our food is being processed to death, they have demonstrated it in scientifically controlled studies.

Dr. Burkitt, who is on Britain's Medical Research Council, has been particularly explicit in his papers on refinement of carbohydrates. In February 1971, he stated to the National (U.S.) Conference on Cancer of the Colon and Rectum that the higher ratio of refined carbohydrates in the American diet has increased the exposure to carcinogens (substances that tend to produce cancer) in the colon and rectum, with a consequent increase in both benign and malignant tumors. Shortly thereafter, he published an article entitled, "The Importance of Fibre in Food," in which he links the removal of the nondigestible fibers from grain and flour to the following illnesses of the so-called "developed" countries: coronary heart disease, cancer of the large bowel, noncancerous tumors in the large intestine, appendicitis, gall bladder disease, diabetes, dental caries, varicose veins, hemorrhoids, deep vein thrombosis, hiatus hernia, and diverticular disease.

Every year the nutrients and vitamins in the average American supermarket diet decrease by a marked percentage due to processing because, in its anxiety to show a profit, the American food industry has lost sight of the fact that it is in the business of providing nutrition, not just empty calories, to the American public. This irresponsibility is then compounded by applying the word "enriched" to heavily refined grain and cereal products. This is worse than nonsense because twenty-four known nutrients are removed and only four are required to be put back for "enrichment." Such a statement deludes the public, which has been lulled to sleep since the Food and Drug Administration gives its blessing to the enrichment rip-off. (See Table on pages 154–155.)

Furthermore, some of the most distinguished nutritionists, who made the excellent recommendation to weight watchers that they "cut down, not out," fall into the trap of condoning this so-called enrichment. Since processing plus enrichment actually "cuts out" a major portion of the vitamins, minerals, and other nutrients of the grain, it seems to us to place the nutritionist in a contradictory position. On the other hand, if the processor were to start with 100 percent whole grain flour and round out the protein by adding wheat germ, soy flour, noninstant skim milk, brewer's yeast, or even lysine, it would not only make sense nutritionally but would justify the use of the word "enriched."

The best solution to this problem is to buy whole grain and cereal products at health food stores. We suggest that the food shopper treat the health food store approach with

GRAIN AND FLOUR CALORIE AND VITAMIN COMPARISON

	Food Energy* or Calories Per Pound	% Protein* by Weight
Minimum FDA requirement for white flour for "enrichment"		—
Unenriched		
Brewer's yeast (debittered)	1284	38.8
Soy flour (full fat)	1910	36.7
Wheat germ (crude)	1647	26.6
Wheat bran (crude)	966	16.0
Rice bran	1252	13.3
Rye flour, dark	1483	16.3
Oats, rolled (uncooked)	1769	14.2
Wheat flour, whole (hard wheats)	1510	13.3
Rice, brown (uncooked)	1633	7.5
Rice, polished (uncooked)	1647	6.7
Wheat flour, white (all purpose)	1651	10.5
Wheat flour, white (cake or pastry)	1651	7.5
Minimum FDA requirement for bread for "enrichment"		—
Bread (2 percent nonfat dry milk added in both cases; no other enrichment)		
Whole wheat	1102	10.5
White	1220	8.7

* All values from *Composition of Foods—Raw, Processed, Prepared*, Agriculture Handbook No. 8, Agricultural Research Service, USDA.

		In Milligrams Per Pound				% Fiber
Thiamine B_1	Riboflavin B_2	Niacin	Iron	Calcium	Potassium**	by Weight
2.0	1.2	16.0	13.0	None	None	None
70.81	19.41	171.9	78.5	953	8,591	1.7
3.85	1.41	9.6	38.1	903	7,530	2.4
9.10	3.09	19.2	42.6	327	3,751	2.5
3.25	1.59	95.3	67.6	540	5,085	9.1
10.25	1.14	135.4	88.0	345	6,781	11.5
2.76	0.98	12.2	20.4	245	3,901	2.4
2.72	0.64	4.5	20.4	240	1,597	1.2
2.49	0.54	19.7	15.0	186	1,678	2.3
1.52	0.24	21.4	7.3	145	971	0.9
0.32	0.12	7.2	3.6	109	417	0.3
0.28	0.21	4.1	3.6	73	431	0.3
0.14	0.14	3.0	2.3	77	431	0.2
1.1	0.7	10.0	8.0	None	None	None
1.17	0.56	12.9	10.4	449	1,238	1.6
0.40	0.36	5.6	3.2	318	386	0.2

The reasons why research is pointing out the need for additional potassium in the
American diet is apparent in the above figures, which show the amount lost in refinement. However, with exercise the need for potassium-rich food is even greater. To
supplement your regular diet, use soy beans, wheat or rice bran, and the much-
maligned blackstrap molasses, which contains 13,277 mg. of potassium per pound.

CEREAL COST
AND NUTRITION COMPARISON

	Size	Low-range Supermarket Prices, February 1976	Protein
Raw wheat germ	20 oz.	.92	26.6% DA
Kellogg's Special K	15 oz.	.99	21.2% m
Old Fashioned Quaker Oats	18 oz.	.59	14.1% m
Oatmeal or rolled oats	18 oz.	.57	14.2% DA
Wheaties	18 oz.	.89	10.6% m
Kellogg's Product 19	12 oz.	.89	10.6% m
Yellow corn meal (refined)	24 oz.	.59	7.1% m
Kellogg's Corn Flakes	18 oz.	.65	7.1% m
Wheatena	22 oz.	.67	14.1% m

m. Manufacturer's figure.
DA. Indicates figures from *Composition of Foods—Raw, Processed, Prepared*, Agriculture Handbook No. 8, Agricultural Research Service, USDA.

common sense. Any theory that extolls one particular food
to the exclusion of others should be suspected. Brown rice,
wheat germ, or seaweed are excellent as parts of our diet,
but to eat any one of them exclusively will undoubtedly result in terminal malnutrition, provided the victim doesn't
die of boredom first.

We want a broad selection of grains and cereals the
way they come on the stalk, *and without chemical additives of any kind!* Highly processed white flour isn't good
enough for animals, vermin, and insects, so they leave it
alone. The milling company can fool us but not the instinc-
tual response of a mouse.

More specific reasons for using whole grain cereals,
breads, and flours are shown in the Table on pages 154–155.

Carbo-hydrate % by Weight	Fat	Cost per Serving[1]	Protein (per ounce by weight)		Calories (per ounce by weight)
			Ounces	Grams	
46.7% DA	10.9% DA	.046	.266 DA	7.5 DA	103 DA
74.1% m	0.0% m	.066[2]	.212 m	6.0 m	110 m
63.5% m	7.1% m	.033	.141 m	4.0 m	110 m
68.2% DA	7.4% DA	.032	.142 DA	4.0 DA	111 DA
81.1% m	3.5% m	.049	.106 m	3.0 m	110 m
84.7% m	0.0% m	.074	.106 m	3.0 m	110 m
74.1% m	3.5% m	.025	.071 m	2.0 m	100 m
88.2% m	0.0% m	.036[3]	.071 m	2.0 m	110 m
74.1% m	3.5% m	.03	.141 m	4.0 m	110 m

. 1 ounce by weight uncooked, equal to approximately 1 cup of cooked cereal or 1 up of dry cereal, except where indicated.
. 1½ cups.
. 1¹/₃ cups.

Note the drop in protein caused by refinement, and the comparison between minimum FDA standards required to advertise white flour and bread as "enriched" and various flours and breads without enrichment.

It can be seen from these comparisons that the parts of the grain that are processed out in refinement are high in the iron and the B vitamins which the FDA says you have to put back in order to use the word "enriched." However, as we have mentioned, many more nutrients come out and usually only four to six go back in. Just like Humpty-Dumpty, once the milling company has fractionated the whole wheat by refinement, "All the king's horses and all the king's men" can't put the wheat kernel together again.

Most commercial dry cereals are so heavily processed

and loaded with sugar that they can only be classified as "junk foods" and their advertising claims are far from truth. The extra trouble of preparing whole grain hot cereals is worth it and, if carefully purchased, will be substantially cheaper. (See Table on pages 156–157.)

In response to a question on normal cholesterol values, in the Consultation Column of the *Medical Tribune,* October 24, 1970, Dr. Richard C. Bozian recommended: ". . . improved whole grain, whole fruit and vegetable intake, and decreased refined carbohydrate intake. We use this program not alone because of its hypocholesterolemic [cholesterol-lowering] effect but because it addresses itself to current life-style errors and constitutes sound health and nutritional practice without risk. Irrespective of lipid [blood fat] changes, patients feel better and promptly."

Apart from the loss of nutrition and the danger of carcinogenicity caused by heavy processing and refinement of grains and cereals, a recent report by Dr. Henry A. Schroeder, of the Dartmouth Medical School's Research Institute, points out that the process of refining flour, sugar, and polished rice increases the cadmium–zinc ratio and that the relative "enrichment" with cadmium during processing is a factor in causing high blood pressure and kidney disorders. This imbalance can be partly offset by adding to your diet the mixture of bran, wheat germ, and brewer's yeast on page 150. It is a good source of zinc.

From the table on page 156 it appears that wheat germ is the best nutritional buy for a breakfast cereal. Mixed half and half with corn meal or rolled oats with some bran added, it gives a delicious hot cereal for about 2½¢ to 3½¢ per serving. Served with skim milk, it contains valuable good-quality protein. To come even close to the same nourishment in a processed packaged cereal, you would have to pay more than double for it, which seems a pretty steep markup just to save a little cooking.

Because of their exceptional nutritional value, nuts and edible seeds deserve to be mentioned separately. It seems that nature sends, along with the germ of life that they contain, a special package of nourishment to give the sprouting plant a good start in its struggle for existence. Thus, seeds generally have high amounts of potassium, magnesium, and phosphorous. Some of them have appreciable amounts of thiamine, niacin, and a good vegetable protein. With this bountiful supply of nutrients, it is unfortunate that they frequently are overlooked or get deliberately strained out in fancy recipes. Our only qualification, while you are losing weight, is to be sure to count their calories, as nuts are loaded with fat. On the other hand, if you have room for them in your calorie count, they are at the top of the list as sources of vegetable protein and minerals.

GROUP 2—DAIRY PRODUCTS
DAILY ALLOWANCE

	Average Calories for Amounts Shown	Average Grams of Protein for Amounts Shown	
1 pint per day of skim milk, buttermilk, low fat milk, or yogurt, in addition to cereal allowance.		Gross Protein	NPU
Alternates: Cheeses (Natural, i.e., not processed) 2 ounces, or Cottage Cheese (creamed) ½ cup	187	15.3	11.8

Unless you are in a very high physical output program or have already reached your correct weight, you are better off with these low-fat products rather than with whole milk. You will then leave yourself more calorie room for a pat of butter or some sour cream or cheese here and there, or can use whole milk or some half-and-half in your coffee. (Buy natural rather than processed cheese, which is made with hydrogenated fat.)

There are also some excellent low-fat yogurts on the market. But look out for the fruit additives; they are loaded with refined-sugar calories and there is usually no way to count their calories. If you can get a good quality cottage cheese, it is excellent for salads and salad dressings, or as a sour cream or butter substitute. Added lemon juice will thin it out and some grated onion will give it zip.

Stay away from dairy substitutes. Most of them are made with coconut oil, which is far more highly saturated than butterfat.

Nature put the butterfat (which is 58 percent saturated fat) and cholesterol in mother's milk and cow's milk for some very good reasons. But nature never intended that we should be as sedentary as we are, which is the real reason why the problem of fats has become so acute, and why most authorities agree on the desirability of the average person cutting down on all fats in the diet. However, once you have reached your correct weight and are on a regular schedule of vigorous exercise, there are studies that suggest that inclusion of a glass or two of whole milk per day with your dairy products is advisable.

GROUP 3—FRUITS

Eat a wide selection of every kind of fruit in its season, fresh; but select some from A, high in Vitamin C, and some from B for other nutrients and variety. During the winter months, order a box of citrus fruits from a reliable supplier at regular intervals. Supplement this with good-quality frozen fruits, and any reasonably priced fresh fruits in the market. Bananas are usually available, and with new methods of mechanical refrigeration excellent apples can be had through the winter.

The dried fruits, apricots, figs, prunes, and raisins, are good, too. They are pleasanter to eat soaked or stewed and are easier on the teeth.

DAILY ALLOWANCE

	Average Calories for Amounts Shown	Average Grams of Protein for Amounts Shown
FRUITS A—HIGH IN VITAMIN C		

Preferably fresh and eaten raw; if not available fresh, use only
    fruits canned without sugars or preservatives.

2 cups per day from any of these combinations	Gross Protein	NPU
Cantaloupe (get the kind with orange-colored flesh)		
Citrus fruits		
Guavas (6 times as much Vitamin C as grapefruit)	153	2.3	0*
Papayas (also high in Vitamin A)		
Persimmons (also high in Vitamin A)		
Strawberries		

Guavas, papayas, and persimmons from subtropical and tropical areas, do provide variety and occasionally are seen in Northern markets.

FRUITS B—FOR OTHER NUTRIENTS AND FOR VARIETY
2 cups per day of these in any combination

Apples, 2 med.
    = approximately 2 cups,
    chopped			

Apricots, 5–6 (high in
    Vitamin A)
    = approximately 2 cups,
    chopped			

Bananas, 2, 6 × 1½ inches
    = approximately 2 cups,
    sliced			

Berries			
Cherries			
Cranberries			

Figs, fresh, 5–6
    = approximately 2 cups,
    chopped
	175	2.1	0*

Grapes			

Peaches, 3 med. (high in
    Vitamin A)
    = approximately 2 cups,
    sliced			

Pears, 2 med. 3 × 2¾ inches
    = approximately 2 cups,
    chopped			

Pineapple, 5–6 slices
    = approximately 2 cups,
    chopped			

Plums, 4, 2 inches in diameter
    = approximately 2 cups,
    sliced			

* Fruit protein is of such low biologic value it is disregarded.

GROUP 4—VEGETABLES

DAILY ALLOWANCE

1½ cups cooked, total per day from a selection of A and B. Average both groups.	*Average Calories for Amounts Shown*	*Average Grams of Protein for Amounts Shown*	
A—FOR VITAMIN A		*Gross Protein*	*NPU*
Beet greens			
Carrots			
Chard, Swiss			
Collards			
Endive and escarole (raw) ½ lb.			
Kale			
Mustard greens			
Peppers (mature, red—five times as much Vitamin C as grapefruit)			
Spinach			
Squash (butternut, or Hubbard, baked)			
Sweet potatoes (baked in skin)			
Turnip greens			
Watercress (raw)			
B—FOR OTHER NUTRIENTS AND FOR VARIETY	80	4.0	2.0
Asparagus			
Beets			
Broccoli			
Celery, 1 large stalk			
Corn, 1 ear, 5 inches long			
Cucumbers			
Green beans			
Onions (raw) young green, 6 small			
Onions			

	Average Calories for Amounts Shown	Average Grams of Protein for Amounts Shown	
		Gross Protein	NPU
Peas*			
Potatoes (baked only)			
Radishes (raw) 5 small			
Red cabbage (raw, it has 50 percent more Vitamin C than grapefruit)			
Tomatoes, raw			

A large salad should be added to your daily menu from the following, which are sometimes known as free vegetables, because they are very low in calories. Besides being delicious, this kind of salad is loaded with vitamins, minerals, and much-needed fiber. But avoid commercial dressings that are made with sugar and hydrogenated oils. Using a cottage cheese or yogurt dressing with onion, blue cheese, and herbs to your taste, it comes to about 150–175 calories including the low-calorie dressing for a good-sized salad: aspara-   163   3.6   0

* These are high in calories, so be sure to count them.

	Average Calories for Amounts Shown	Average Grams of Protein for Amounts Shown
		Gross Protein *NPU*

gus, bean sprouts, beet greens, broccoli, carrots (raw only), cauliflower, celery, chicory, Chinese peapods, cucumbers, endive and escarole, French-type string beans, kale, lettuce, mushrooms, mustard greens, okra, peppers, radishes, red cabbage, sauerkraut, spinach, Swiss chard, tomatoes (raw only), turnip greens, watercress, and zucchini.

Most of the above vegetables are available all year, but if you are fortunate enough to have a patch of ground that gets some sunlight, add a summer garden. Your own vegetables, including herbs, will enhance meals with flavor you just can't buy.

In winter, buy fresh vegetables in the market when you can live with the prices and supplement with good-quality frozen vegetables. Avoid tricky packaging and "butter added"; you'll pay more than it's worth.

Eat as many vegetables as possible raw. When you do cook, cook as lightly as possible, or steam. Save the water for soups. Dumping the water can waste as much as 35 percent of the vitamins and minerals in the vegetable.

Soybeans

Soybeans have so many good qualities that no one is sure where to put them in a diet program, but as a legume they belong with the vegetables. They are a rich source of the B-complex vitamins, as well as calcium, potassium, and phosphorous, and the fat they contain is mostly unsaturated. Their NPU is among the highest of the vegetable sources; although not as high as the protein from milk, eggs, and meat, on an uncooked comparison they contain twice as much protein by weight as beef.

In bean form or as flour for bread, they are an excellent and inexpensive part of a good diet. You may have to go to a specialty store for them and consult the cookbook on how to handle them. But, on both counts, they are worth the trouble.

GROUP 5—MEATS

One of these twice a week: beef, lamb, veal. Try to buy meat, not fat. Prime and choice meats are very fatty meats—so-called "marbled." This traditional standard of "high quality" is not sound nutrition. Devotion to the huge steak with French fries as a marvelous meal and a great treat is ingrained in the American culture. But, especially for a sedentary person, it is indigestible, over a long period dangerous, and grossly uneconomical because you pay dearly for the marbling and the outside fat, which run off in the cooking. However, flank or beef shoulder cuts are delicious and have far less fat. You will get a third to a half more protein for the cut you buy and they cost less than prime or choice steak. If you could tell the different grades of meat, it would be better to buy "Good" (medium or thin class for veal) of the cuts shown below, avoiding Prime or Choice. However, it is difficult to know what to buy from the confusing array of cuts, so the only way to select seems to be by using a little common sense. A porterhouse or T-bone at $2.79 per pound sounds good, but is easily 40–45 percent fat and bone. A flank or round, cut for London broil, at $2.19 to $2.49 with 6–12 percent fat and no bone is a far better buy. As a guide, the following cuts are generally lower in fat content and higher in protein:

DAILY ALLOWANCE

Trim all fat. All portions are 4 ounces raw, two times per week	*Average Calories for 4-Ounce Portions*	*Average Grams of Protein for 4-Ounce Portions*	
		Gross Protein	*NPU*
BEEF			
Flank			
Arm chuck			
Round			
Hamburger (buy lean meat only, see it ground at the store; most commercial hamburger has 10–20 percent fat added so avoid it)			
LAMB	163	23.4	15.2
Leg			
Loin			
VEAL (Thin Class)			
Chuck			
Foreshank			
Liver			
Loin			
Round with rump			

Smoked meats should be avoided, if possible. Occasionally, they aren't going to hurt a healthy person. However, they are processed with chemicals that have been connected with lung cancer. This is probably a controversial issue as the information is limited, but it's better to stick to fresh meats.

Pork should be considered in a separate category. First, the leaner the pork, the better for you. Secondly, and more important, unless you are willing to cook pork with a meat thermometer, as described in any good cookbook, it would be better to forget it. If overcooked, the meat is ruined nutritionally and, if undercooked, you and your family risk trichinal infection. Don't assume that because it has been "inspected" the pork is free of this disease. In any case, with these precautions, pork can be included.

GROUP 6—FISH

There has been so much discussion about mercury and pesticides in fish that it should at least be mentioned. Generally, some very contradictory reports have come out, but it seems clear that shellfish and the smaller less predatory fish, which are not so far up on the food chain, tend to have less of these contaminants. However, avoid raw or incompletely cooked shellfish; it isn't worth the risk of hepatitis from polluted waters. Fish is tremendously important in the diet. It is very high in excellent quality protein. The fat is largely unsaturated, and to cut down or out would be a great detriment to the diet.

DAILY ALLOWANCE

All portions 5 ounces raw, 3 times per week (Fresh when possible, broiled or baked only)	Average Calories for 5-Ounce Portion	Average Grams of Protein for 5-Ounce Portion	
		Gross Protein	NPU
Bass, black, sea			
Bass, smallmouth and largemouth			
Bass, striped			
Bluefish			
Carp			
Clams			
Cod			
Crab			
Flatfishes (flounder, fluke, and sole)			
Grouper (all kinds)	134	25.3	20.2
Haddock			
Halibut			
Lobster			
Ocean perch (redfish)			
Oysters			
Red and gray snapper			
Scallops			
Sea bass			
Shrimp			
Tuna*			
Weakfish			

(Mackerel, salmon, sardines, and shad omitted as they range from 200–300 calories per portion)

* Tuna is high on the food chain and has been reported to have more than a safe level of mercury.

GROUP 7—POULTRY AND EGGS

Chicken is relatively inexpensive and high in protein, and contains less saturated fat than beef or lamb. The problem is in buying it. Most market chickens are raised on wire, are confined and overfed so that they have very little flavor. Capons are even worse; they taste flat and are mostly caponized with a hormone. Don't buy them or knowingly eat them. If you know a farmer whose chickens are raised outside on the ground, you will do better to patronize him even if it costs more. Guinea hen is also a good bird if available. Poultry should be included three times a week. Include in this category an occasional piece of game that comes your way. Upland birds, pheasant, grouse, woodcock, etc., tend to be low in fat and very high in protein. Although waterfowl have more fat, you probably won't have them often enough to make any difference. In any case, they provide an enjoyable change in the routine.

Ask the farmer who sells you the chickens raised on the range if he has fertile eggs—brown, white, or spotted. (Recently some health food stores have started to handle these eggs.) They have more flavor and the chances are they have a better mineral content resulting from the bird's free choice of foods on the range. There are 250–255 mgs. of cholesterol in the egg yolk and some nutritionists advise restricting them in the diet, especially for people over forty. On the other hand, certain studies indicate that reduction of dietary cholesterol sparks a feedback mechanism that causes the body to manufacture more cholesterol, creating a stalemate situation. In any case, eggs are an excellent source of protein, Vitamin A, and minerals. So, once on a vigorous exercise program, four a week is a good compromise.

Don't be misled into using powdered eggs in any form, even for cooking or baking. In most heat-dried egg products the cholesterol in the yolk has become crystallized. Crystalline cholesterol is an unstable substance that can oxidize to form other compounds that damage the linings of arteries. Dried eggs are frequently used by commercial bakers in bread and cakes, and also in dried soups, so these should be avoided as well.

Vary your selection from among the following:

DAILY ALLOWANCE

All poultry portions 4 ounces raw, 3 times per week	Average Calories for 4-Ounce Portion	Average Grams of Protein for 4-Ounce Portion	
		Gross Protein	NPU
CHICKEN			
Fryers: Breast			
Drumstick			
Thigh			
Wing			
Roasters: Whole Bird			
Liver			
GUINEA HEN	165	22.8	15.2
Whole bird			
TURKEY			
Young bird			
(24 weeks and under)			
Medium bird			
(26–32 weeks)			
EGGS			
(4 per week)			
1 medium, large,	84	6.5	6.1
or extra large			

SUMMARY OF CALORIES AND PROTEIN
IN TOTAL DIET

| | DAILY AVERAGE OF WEEKLY TOTALS | | | TOTALS PER WEEK | | |
| | *Grams of Protein* | | | *Grams of Protein* | | |
	Calories	Gross Protein	NPU	Calories	Gross Protein	NPU
Regular diet from the seven food groups	1,616	92.1	55.6	11,310	644.8	389.2
Extras: Butter on bread and vegetables, sour cream on potatoes, and miscellaneous	350	0	0	2,450	0	0
Whole milk for cereal, coffee, tea, etc.	160	8.0	6.6	1,120	56.0	46.2
	2,126	100.1	62.2	14,880	700.8	435.4

A varied selection at each meal from these seven groups for an absolute minimum of three meals a day will give you a good balanced diet and should generally eliminate the need for supplemental vitamins. In some cases, extra B-complex and C may be desirable in connection with high output exercise programs. Whether or not to recommend a one-a-day all-round vitamin and mineral pill is up to your doctor. Since extra unneeded doses of A and D can cause toxicity, the amount of these you take should be prescribed by your doctor. In any case, many of the foods listed above have plenty of Vitamin A, and since milk and certain other foods usually have added Vitamin D, he may tell you that you don't need any supplement of these vitamins.

Select one or more foods from each of the seven food groups every day and go for contrasting color patterns. They are aesthetically appealing and, whether nature designed it that way or whether it is a coincidence, contrasting color patterns tend to balance the diet. For example,

Stewed or fricassee chicken
Mashed potatoes
Buttered noodles
White bread

is unappetizing and unbalanced.

Instead, try:

Broiled chicken—with a sprinkle of chopped parsley or tarragon and a dash of paprika.

Baked potato—Leave it in the jacket; open and top it with cottage cheese and chives.

On the side—Salad of sliced tomatoes, fresh raw spinach, watercress, and chopped radishes; garnished with raw carrot sticks and sprinkled with marjoram or mixed salad herbs. Use a dressing made with yogurt and a small amount of grated onion and blue cheese.

Slice of whole wheat bread

Glass of skim milk or buttermilk

It's not much more trouble, if any, but what a difference!

Select from these within your calorie range and subject to weekly limits and minima:

Breakfast

1 cup fruit from Group A
1 cup cereal with bran mixture

1 slice whole grain bread (wheat, rye, oatmeal, corn, soya, etc.) with 2 level teaspoons of butter, maximum.

Fish, or egg (subject to limits)

8 ounces skim milk, buttermilk, or low fat milk

Coffee or tea (see limit, page 176). If you wish, dissolve instant in 2 ounces very hot water and fill with warm skim milk from the 8 ounces.

Lunch

1 cup broth (avoid heavy, creamed, or greasy soups)

Poultry, fish, or ½ cup cottage cheese

Salad from Groups A and B—try one made with Boston lettuce, endive, or escarole, sliced raw mushrooms, chopped raw zucchini, chopped raw asparagus tips, ½ red sweet pepper sliced in thin strips, two chopped green olives. Use a dressing made with a combination of cottage cheese and buttermilk or yogurt, seasoned with curry and a small amount of English mustard or capers and soya sauce.

2 slices whole grain bread or seven grain bread (available in some health food stores) with two level teaspoons of butter.

8 ounces skim milk, buttermilk, or yogurt

Before Dinner Canapés

Have your drink, if it is your custom, but count it. If it isn't, join the others with bouillon, clamato, or tomato juice "on-the-rocks."

Cauliflower bits

Carrots (raw)

Celery

Cherry tomatoes

Radishes

Cottage cheese dip (easy on the salt)

Dinner

Chicken, fish, or meat

Small baked potato (eat the jacket), topped with cottage
cheese and chives, or ½ cup baked beans* once a
week.

¾ cup green or yellow vegetable from Group A

¾ cup vegetable from Groups A or B

1 slice whole wheat bread

1 cup fruit from Group A

Bran mixture (with fruit or milk)

8 ounces skim milk, low-fat milk, or yogurt

Cooking

Eat as many vegetables raw as possible. Contrary to popular belief, such vegetables as zucchini, asparagus, cauliflower, and broccoli can be eaten raw in salads or as
snacks. Those that must be cooked should be steamed or
cooked otherwise as lightly as possible. Save the juices and
serve them with the vegetables or in a soup.

Bake, broil, or roast meats. Where oil is needed, brush
with a light vegetable oil (safflower, corn, or soy, in that
order). Fried foods should be eliminated from the diet, especially deep fat fried. The hard, saturated, boiled-over oil
that is generally used at high temperatures to fry French-
fried potatoes, doughnuts, and fried fish and chicken is
indigestible and dangerous. An occasional helping won't
kill you, which you eat to avoid embarrassment with an un-
informed hostess, but, generally, stay away from fried

* Use soy beans. See: *The Joy of Cooking,* Irma S. Rombauer and Marion
Rombauer Becker (Indianapolis: Bobbs-Merrill, Revised Edition, 1975).

foods which are clearly unhealthful and, through laziness and convenience, have become built into our pattern of eating. Certainly at home it has no basis either on the grounds of economy or nutrition.

There are many excellent nutrition-oriented books available today with sound advice on cooking, among which we recommend:

Eat Well and Stay Well, Ancel and Margaret Keys (Garden City, New York: Doubleday, 2nd Edition, 1963).

The Joy of Cooking, Irma S. Rombauer and Marion Rombauer Becker (Indianapolis: Bobbs-Merrill, Revised Edition, 1975).

What You Need to Know About Food & Cooking for Health, Lawrence E. Lamb, M.D. (New York: Viking Press, 1973).

Low-Fat Cookery, Evelyn S. Stead and Gloria K. Warren (New York: McGraw-Hill, 1956-59).

Coffee and Tea

In limited quantities, two cups a day total of coffee or tea probably won't do a healthy person any harm; preferably, the last cup at lunch time. Coffee and tea are pleasant and sociable, and provide a mild stimulation. However, if they make you uncomfortable or give you indigestion, maybe they are not for you. Anyone is probably better off without them.

The Alcohol Culture

Here is the way it works: A man and a woman stopped at an expensive restaurant in Connecticut. Typical of the "alcohol culture" in which we have been brought up, they walked in slowly, a couple in their late forties. Confident, well dressed, and each 30 pounds overweight, they nodded to the waitress as she indicated a table. The man had thick, rimmed glasses and a white, jowly expression. The woman had iron-gray hair and a lined face, the hardness ill-concealed by her set smile.

When they were seated, the waitress said snidely: "The usual, with the olive?"

The act and the ceremony followed. First they pretended to debate whether they would have one or not; then they would. Finally, the drinks arrived, two on the stem, like little beaded flower pots, iridescent, with the meaningless olive rolling like a dead tadpole in the strong alcohol.

As the third pair of drinks arrived, the couple decided to order their marbled steaks and baked potatoes drenched with butter. By the time they arrived, both the man and the woman were glassy-eyed and were mouthing their words. They were at the stage where they would only dimly remember the dinner, let alone enjoy the $30 meal while they were eating it.

Sadly enough, this ritual has become so built into our mores that we think we can't get along without it. And it all started a long time ago, because alcohol in one form or another has been consumed by humans for thousands of years. There's not much to be said for it except that a glass of cool beer can be pleasant on a hot day, as can an orange or lemonade. Also, a good wine at dinner is a pleasure. So, in moderation, let's go along.

Here are two tough rules: (1) no alcohol at least 12 hours before hard exercise since alcohol will interfere with the delivery of oxygen to the cells and impair performance; (2) after hard exercise, don't drink alcohol in any form for at least two to four hours, depending on the degree of exertion.

That alcohol, after high stress exercise of long duration, is an insult to the cardiovascular system is supported by medical and scientific opinion. The blocking or sludging effect in the capillaries has been well documented by Professor Melvin H. Knisely, and Drs. Herbert A. Moskow and Raymond C. Pennington at the Medical University of South Carolina.

Since oxygen is vital to the removal of waste products resulting from hard physical work, alcohol seriously hinders the repair and recovery of muscular tissue. Even a person in top physical condition who has played hard tennis for two hours should replace all the fluid lost (which could be two to three quarts) with water and some dissolved salt (see Chapter 11, page 191) and have it settled down before he even thinks about alcohol. Actually, if he's in such good shape, he's probably not that interested in alcohol anyway.

Smoking

Although tobacco is certainly not a food, comments on it seem appropriate as a sequel to alcohol. So far we have only referred generally to smoking as a serious detriment to health. However, as former smokers we have experienced it subjectively as well as objectively and can say that no one feels as much antipathy to it as some one does who has kicked the habit. Now, we can't understand how we were once so inconsiderate as to subject others to it, because for a nonsmoker a thick, smoky atmosphere is sheer misery.

The number of smokers in the United States is now below 25 percent of the population, down from 44 percent just a few years ago, so people are getting the message, which is a pretty frightening one. Despite the platitudes of the tobacco companies, which are nothing other than dishonest, cigarettes are proven killers. If inhaled, cigars and pipes are the same and even without inhaling they can cause cancer of the lips and mouth.

Dr. Kenneth H. Cooper has mounted under glass in his office in Dallas two pieces of human lung. The healthy specimen is pink and the unhealthy smoker's lung has thick, black deposits clogging up the passageways very much like the infamous "black lung" suffered by coal miners.

Our position on smoking is shared by an increasing majority who aren't quite as vocal on the subject. Although this will probably make us unpopular with a few of our friends who still smoke, it has to be said because this is a book on health and, of all the habits and customs that are legally and socially tolerated in our society, smoking is the most damaging to health.

Sugar and Artificial Sweeteners

In a sound diet program, elimination of refined flour and sugar in any form is essential, especially in all commercial baked goods, candy, and sweet desserts. These are "empty calories," so take carbohydrates in the whole grain breads and cereals, fruits, and sweet vegetables (carrots, tomatoes, etc.). Some say artificial sweeteners create a dependency and a compensatory attitude, but others feel that the saccharine-based ones are pleasant and helpful. Certainly, for over fifty years, they have demonstrated that in moderate quantities they are harmless. We suspect that the cyclamates are probably harmless as well. However, it won't hurt to stay away from them until the Department of Health, Education, and Welfare and the Food and Drug Administration reverse their original position and give them final clearance.

10 | The Weight

Merriam-Webster's Third International Dictionary gives fourteen definitions of weight. Here are some of the more familiar ones: In a figurative sense, "Mr. Johnson carries a lot of weight on the committee"; or, in a relative sense, "the weight of the astronauts on the moon was one-sixth of their weight on earth"; or, specifically, "when the Smiths checked in at the airport, their luggage was 15 pounds overweight."

Perhaps it's just as well the airlines don't have a charge for people who are overweight. For example: the airline representative would say, "Step on the scales, please, Mr. Smith." Mr. Smith looks furious but steps on the scales. His height is quickly checked, he gives his age, and the man says, "Mr. Smith, you're 15 pounds over the weight allowance. It's a dollar a pound, you know, so that will be $15 more, please." We'll leave Mr. Smith's reaction to your imagination, because what one weighs is a highly personal matter, and people can be very touchy about it. Some people won't even tell you what they weigh, until they start to lose seriously. Then it comes out as a matter of pride in their accomplishment.

But apart from this sensitivity, the airline would have a tough time telling Mr. Smith what he should weigh. Maybe he is a professional football player and the 15 pounds are all muscle, or he is a big man with a large amount of lean body mass, big frame and heavy bones, all of which could easily weigh 15 pounds more than a tall, thin man with a light frame. However, to understand why these differences in weight exist, let's have another look at the somatotypes, or body types, that were reviewed in Chapter 1 in relation to weight.

William Sheldon's *Atlas of Men* shows pictures of 1,175 different men with varying types of builds. While they shade from one type to another, there are three basic ones to consider.

As described in Chapter 1, the endomorph is round and roly-poly, has an even temperament, puts on weight as fat easily and has a very hard time taking it off. He really has to work at it as his body tends to run to a high percentage of fat. If you recognize the type in yourself, you'll just have to cut down on fats in your diet, especially in those prime and choice meats, reduce the bread and potato portions by one-half, and fill up with citrus fruits and leafy vegetables, at least until you reach your optimum weight.

The mesomorph is aggressive and has heavy bones

and muscles, which will make him weigh more at a given height. He has to look out too, since an over-fat meso-morph seems to be prone later on to heart attacks and strokes. He needs the same diet restrictions as the endo-morph and should work on the light, fast exercises to build flexibility and cardiopulmonary endurance.

The ectomorph is the thin, lean individual who tends to be introspective and who seems to be able to eat enor-mous amounts of food and never get fat. Studies indicate that he moves more than other types, which helps to burn it up. There is also a difference in metabolism. He has no need to restrict his food intake but he does need to keep fit to avoid respiratory ailments. Many great runners tend generally to be ectomorphic types.

Besides the different meanings of the word "weight," the amount each individual has of fat, bone, muscle, and other lean tissue and organs varies according to individual types and characteristics. While we were given a certain size heart, stomach, and other organs, and can take good care of them by keeping in shape, we can't do much to change their basic size or weight. Therefore, we have to give our attention to the dramatic changes we can make in reducing fat and increasing bone and muscle with a combi-nation of diet and exercise. The amount of bone added would be extremely small in terms of overall weight, but it is very significant from the standpoint of structural strength. Furthermore, a fat person will usually take off a lot more weight in fat than he puts on in bone and muscle, but since muscle weighs nearly 1½ times as much as fat there are a few people who can go from fat to fit with rela-tively little change in weight. The methods of determining how much fat they lost and how much muscle they gained is a very complicated procedure, but here is an extreme comparison of a sedentary man with an active fit and muscular man:

BREAKDOWN OF COMPONENT WEIGHTS

	Sedentary Man	*Active and Fit Man*
Fat	49.8 lbs.	19.9 lbs.
Muscle	23.2 lbs.	61.0 lbs.
Other (bone, organs, fluid, lean tissue mass, etc.)	102.0 lbs.	94.1 lbs.
Weight	175.0 lbs.	175.0 lbs.

There are some confusing factors in weight loss or gain. Weight can be lost from inactivity, which once happened to a man we know, who was on an extended business trip during which his exercise program had to be curtailed. Combined with poor diet and lack of sleep, he lost from 1 to 2 pounds a week, and yet there was no apparent dimensional change. It was just that fat replaced muscle and he felt exhausted in the bargain. More recently, he went away for two weeks and was able to keep his exercise program close to normal. His weight stayed the same and he felt well and enjoyed the trip.

The next source of confusion is fluid balance, which is the most misunderstood factor in body weight. An example is the woman (125 lbs.) who exclaimed: "I gained 3 pounds over the long weekend; how will I ever get it off?" To gain those 3 pounds in fat, she would have had to eat an extra 3,600 calories a day (during the three-day weekend) over and above her daily maintenance requirement of 1,875 calories, or a total of 5,475 calories a day! This is an impossibility unless she was stuffed through a tube like Strasbourg geese. What she did was pick up some extra fluid, which undoubtedly disappeared through her kidneys in a few days when she got back to her normal routine. In fact, a long brisk walk on Monday and Tuesday could have set things right.

Disappointment, as well as confusion, often comes with some of the "high-protein" diets, which, for a while, act metabolically as a diuretic. There is an immediate weight loss due to loss of water and the dieter, innocent and deluded, is delighted until the effect is dissipated and the fluid goes back where it belongs. Now the dieter, who is puzzled and frustrated, must sooner or later forget about these trick diets and learn to cut down, not out, and to step up his or her activity.

In an effort to avoid confusion over water balance, many weight-reducing programs advise weighing yourself only once a week. We don't agree, because you may catch a high day or a low day, which is even more confusing. If you weigh every day you'll get used to the fluid-balance swing and once familiar with it, it won't bother you. Monday morning can be high with a load of food and drink not yet assimilated from the weekend. Usually Thursday or Friday morning is the low point.

Careful weighing before and after very strenuous exercise is advisable also in order to become familiar with the fluid loss. The need for replacement with water and salt is discussed in Chapters 8 and 11.

Actual Weight Loss

The actual reduction in the weight that you want to lose will occur on an average basis over a period of weeks. If you start a program of weight control through exercise and diet on a Monday, you may lose the water balance in the first few days. You should write down your daily weights (or graph them if you are so inclined) and the first reduction will look nice on paper. As mentioned earlier, it is a good idea to get used to these fluctuations, but don't depend on them. Instead, take the average of the first week and the average of the second and compare them.

Another phenomenon is the plateau effect. The average may stay the same and not move for two or three weeks. Then suddenly one morning it's down a pound or two. You'll probably recognize it when it's the real thing, because the reading will be in new low ground where you haven't been in months or years. That's a thrill, and a very important one, because it renews the determination and buoys up the flagging spirit.

Especially at this point, we would advise keeping it to yourself. Because if you announce publicly, "I'm down to so and so," your weight might bound up again for one reason or another and then you'll be embarrassed when someone says, "How much are you down to now?" It's much better to wait until a friend you haven't seen for a while bursts out, "Hey, haven't you lost some weight?" Then be casual, "Oh, a little, just being careful, you know," and change the subject.

How you handle it from there on is up to you. We can only caution you that it's not a subject to dwell on with friends. If they are not on a program themselves, they get bored and feel guilty very quickly. Also, from the friend who has a diet of his own, you can get drawn into this kind of discussion. He says, "You say you lost 5 pounds on that thing you're on? Well, how about this? My wife and I went on this diet we got out on the coast where you drink cream, avoid skim milk, and eat lots of bacon for breakfast and, you know what? I lost 17 pounds in three weeks." At this point, if you're smart, you'll say, "Great! Aren't you lucky to have such a good diet?" Then get off the subject as soon as you can. But make a mental note and see what's happened to his weight and the cream and bacon diet in six months. What is most important is not to get discouraged or enticed when you hear that kind of story, because the woods are full of them. It is obvious that your friend has several factors in that 17 pounds; a large loss of fluid, some exaggeration, plus a difference in scales or clothing. To lose 17 pounds of actual fat in three weeks, your friend, who weighed 190, would have had to do the following: reduce his intake to 1,400 calories a day; remain normally active, plus jog for an hour and a half every day at 6½ mph, or a total of 215 miles. We have a strange feeling he didn't do it.

METHODS OF WEIGHT DETERMINATION
(Besides the Scale)

Skinfold Measurement

Doctors use a caliper designed to exert a constant pressure to measure the thickness of a fold of skin in back of your upper arm (triceps). If you are not obese, this should measure between ¼ and ½ inch. This can best be done by your doctor, but if you want to get a rough idea at home, lightly grip the skin behind your upper arm between the thumb and forefinger. If you feel a thickness of about one-quarter inch or less, you're doing fine. If it's more, you have some fat to lose.

There are other methods for precise determination of

body fat, but they are difficult and can only be done in a lab, so let's go to a good, old-fashioned way of telling.

Tape Measure

For men, the key measurement is around the waist, at the natural indentation, if there is one, standing erect, stomach firm but not sucked in. The proper measurement for you depends on your height and general build. Here are some averages: U.S. Air Force trainees, 30.3 inches; Air Force pilots (older), 32.9 inches; general population (older), 36.6 inches. So it seems clear that the general male population carries nearly 4 inches more fat around the middle than those Air Force pilots. Since these studies were done some years ago, the difference today is probably even more drastic, as the civilian population gets fatter every year and the Air Force is probably in even better shape as a result of aerobic exercise programs initiated in 1966 and 1967 by Dr. Kenneth H. Cooper, then colonel, USAF-MC. In any event, if you protrude at all, it's undoubtedly some fat and some bad posture, and the exercises in Chapters 6 to 8 will help both. Keep a record of the original waist measurement and watch it periodically as it goes down.

Women should measure waists, top of thighs and hips and keep a record of all three. As an example, here are some average waist measurements:

WAF Basic Trainees	25.9 inches
WACs and Army Nurses	26.5 inches
Working Women	28.8 inches
General population (older)	33.1 inches

These averages show that women not in the service but in the general population put on over 7 inches of flab as

they get older. This happens at an older age than men probably because when mom is chasing those kids she doesn't
put it on. But it does go on later. This is all the more reason
to keep track of your measurements. Marjorie Craig, in her
21 Day Shape-Up Program for Men and Women suggests a
total of twelve measurements and gives an extremely comprehensive series of exercises, which will keep them all in
the proper dimensions. Miss Craig, however, has the objective of aesthetic appearance, and since this book is
aimed at cardiopulmonary fitness and general health, we
are only suggesting the three measurements above to tell
the basic story.

Walking and running will make you slim and trim, and
give the best possible appearance that nature ever intended
for your particular figure and legs. Women should not be
concerned that exercises and running will make their
muscles stand out. It's true that almost anyone's muscles
will stand out in a snapshot taken when they are in extreme
contraction, but not when relaxed. Subject to their natural
endowment, women runners have beautiful legs.

HOW TO DECIDE
WHAT YOU SHOULD WEIGH

If you were in pretty good shape at high school graduation
and not too plump, it's a significant weight if you can remember it.

At about age 25 most men and women have probably
been working full time or at least part time for some years.
Usually the man has put on a tire around his waist. He has
had his pants let out and his jacket is getting tight across the
back, but not from muscle.

Now, the lower weight of high school graduation or age 25 is your upper limit for life, and, as you get older your weight should come down somewhat from that limit. The amount depends on how fit you are, but unless you are tremendously fit with hard, wiry muscles, you would be better off 10–15 pounds below it.

Life Insurance Tables

These tables have been used as guides for many years and have caused more confusion than enlightenment about weight. If you are a doctor or a physiologist and know how to do a somatotype rating of your subject and can do a skin-fold test and a lot of calculation, the tables may help. However, at this stage of scientific knowledge about body composition, these tables are a myth that these authors have no desire to perpetuate.

Decreasing Emphasis on Weight as Your Program Progresses Due to Homeostasis

We have described the tendency of the body to maintain the status quo. If you get to the correct weight, stay fit, and if you understand homeostasis (the tendency of the body to maintain things as they are), it can save you a lot of bother, because the odd splurge off your diet doesn't do anything that can't be straightened out the next week. It's as if by coming back to your program the little gland that guides this destiny knows you mean it and pardons you for your indiscretion. But splurge for a week or more and the gland says, "I can't trust this character," and up goes your fat and down comes the muscle. Sometimes the splurge doesn't show as a weight increase right away; sometimes it shows as a slight weight loss if you lose muscle, which weighs nearly 1½ times as much as fat.

If you keep at the program, however, the weight will swing up and down from day to day with the fluid balance, but the average will stay the same. As you exercise more, your appetite will indicate very accurately how much you should eat; in fact the fullness signal will be so strong that it will be almost impossible to ignore it. Then you will have really reached a balance where you will scarcely have to think about it, as it will take care of itself.

11 | Fluid and Electrolyte* Management in High-Stress Physical Exercise

Anyone who goes beyond the basic 2-mile running program described in Chapter 8 should become familiar with fluid and electrolyte management in high-stress exercise.

Although excellent studies on sweating and physical activity were done as early as the 1930s by Harvard physiologist David B. Dill, little of it was known to coaches and athletes, often with tragic incidents, many of them unnecessary in the light of present knowledge.

As an example of a potentially dangerous situation,

---

* The body fluid salts in solution, which include sodium, potassium, magnesium, calcium and others as cations; and chloride, sulfate, phosphate, et al., as anions (limited definition).

one of the authors recalls a school football game on a very warm day (about 80–85° F.) in 1929, in which he played the full four quarters. He weighed, stripped, 192 before the game and 178 afterwards. There were strong prohibitions against drinking water during the game (it would give you cramps, cotton mouth, etc.), so he sneaked only a few swallows. Added salt was unknown. Other teammates had similar losses and it was probably just plain luck and good physical condition that none of the players on either team had a serious incident of heat illness. Not surprisingly, he recalls feeling extremely poorly for the next two days.

With proper management such a weight loss would not be allowed to occur. For example, during the last hour before the game each player should have drunk up to a quart of fluid containing proper electrolytes (see pages 207–210) in solution. The amount taken should be based on individual tolerances determined in prior practice. To avoid possible discomfort, the player should empty his bladder just before the game, and during it take drinks of 6–8 ounces every 10–15 minutes, coming as close to total replacement as possible. At the very extreme no player should probably lose more than 2½ percent of total body weight, in which case he will feel and perform far better. A loss of 3 percent or over will cause a serious decrease in bodily function.

There is much research behind these conclusions and it is vital for coaches and athletes to understand that fact so proper procedures can be used in training.

First, let us look at the symptoms and effects of heat and dehydration illness so they can be recognized.

Heat illness in its first stages is generally called heat exhaustion. It is characterized by one or more of these symptoms: blurred vision, shortness of breath, muscle cramps, dizziness, faintness, palpitation, and extremely rapid but weak pulse, accompanied by headache and rectal temperatures 2–4° above normal. The individual will still be sweating profusely. Upon recognition by the coach or athlete of any of these symptoms alone or in combination, all activity should cease. The individual should then be taken immediately to a cool place and sponged off with cool water. If he is not too nauseated, he should sip slowly a cool (never cold, see page 196) electrolyte solution.

If prolonged, this condition becomes heat stroke, which is far more serious and demands immediate medical attention. Every athlete and sportsman should be familiar with the symptoms of heat stroke and know how to prevent them. Above all, he must know and respect his own limitations, because the penalties are too severe to risk. Heat stroke differs from heat exhaustion in the following ways: instead of a pallid skin and profuse sweating the skin becomes flushed, hot, and dry. Pulse is rapid and strong and rectal temperature is higher than 4° above normal. Muscles will be flaccid and there is frequently delirium and coma. If the condition continues to the point of cardiopulmonary collapse, the skin will have become pallid and the athlete is very ill indeed.

Until the doctor arrives the victim should be moved to a cool place and sponged with cold water. If he shows any loss of consciousness, no attempt should be made to have him drink the electrolyte solution. In any case he probably wouldn't keep enough down to do any good and vomiting would aggravate the problem. The time within which he gets medical treatment is critical, because at this point the victim is in extreme danger of irreversible damage to his body tissues or even death.

The technical details of what actually happens under

these conditions are best described by Dr. John P. Merrill, Director of the Cardiovascular Section at Peter Bent Brigham Hospital in Boston, who says: "By dehydration we imply not only loss of water, as the word suggests, but more important, loss of electrolyte and water. Severe, acute, or prolonged loss of electrolyte and water from the gastrointestinal tract or skin may impair renal dynamics [kidney functioning] to the point where parenchymatous [essential kidney tissue] damage occurs on the basis of ischemia [deficient blood supply due to inadequate inflow of arterial blood]. This damage, once established cannot be immediately reversed by the repair of the fluid and electrolyte deficit."

Seasonal Factors in Heat Illness and How to Avoid It

Hot weather or high humidity creates the risk of heat illness, but in combination the danger is the greatest. Hot, dry weather demands ample fluid intake of a dilute electrolyte solution. Due to the rapid evaporation of sweat, there is an efficient cooling effect. However, in hot, humid weather evaporation is very slow and there is profuse sweating without efficient cooling, hence the danger is increased. Athletes training throughout the summer must adopt a careful program employing preexercise drinks as well as during and afterwards.

Clearly, the greatest exposure to heat exhaustion and heat stroke occurs with sudden hot days in spring, going south for any reason, and hotter than usual days in summer. It can become critical with school and college athletes in early season training due to warm autumn weather and the poorer condition of the individual. Those who have not been training should be brought along very gradually, and in about three weeks should be acclimatized to heat and rigorous training. (In general, acclimatization means the physiological adjustment of the individual to a new temperature, climate, or environment. More specifically, in rigorous training in heat, the body's response in acclimatization is that the sodium chloride content in sweat becomes more dilute. However, the individual hangs on to the sodium chloride at the expense of a greater loss of potassium. Hence the need for electrolyte balance in fluid intake.)

Every effort should be made to have the athlete avoid the long summer layoff and being catapulted into a program of violent exercise. Instead, athletes should be urged to run in the off-season a minimum of 5 to 6 miles a day at seven-to-eight minute miles or better, five days a week, with weight training and calisthenics as a supplement to the running. While coaches may not get 100 percent compliance, the highly motivated athlete will train, and the difference in his condition will be so startling that the point should soon become evident to the others.

In training or competition, fluid and electrolyte requirements should be estimated in advance to ensure that athletes drink amounts as near as possible to 90 percent of gross weight loss (GWL = net loss + weight of fluid drunk during the activity). This requires discipline and the cooperation of the athlete, because he must mark down his weight stripped before and after exercise. A system should be devised to keep a record of the amount consumed (use 6- or 8-ounce cups) so that a net and gross loss can be computed.

As an example, a 175-pound athlete about to take a strenuous one-hour workout in 75° heat (estimated loss 4 pounds) should drink four 8-ounce glasses of water with appropriate electrolytes in the correct solution, depending on tolerance, spread over the half-hour to hour immediately preceding the workout. The electrolyte solution should then be taken throughout the workout at a minimum of 6–8 ounces every 15 minutes. Thus, with three fluid breaks during the workout, plus the preevent fluid, he will have consumed 1¾ quarts, or roughly 90 percent of the 4-pound loss.

Both plain water and electrolyte solution to suit the tolerance of the individual should be available at frequent periods, or continuously when the sport permits. *No ice water!* Dr. Lawrence E. Lamb, Professor of Medicine at Baylor, in his book *Your Heart and How to Live With It* (p. 148), warns against drinking cold fluids immediately after (or during) hard exercise. A drink with a temperature of 65° will have a cooling effect of more than 30° as compared to body temperature. This is a sufficient differential. However, 50° is too much and may cause a shock. He cites cases of two normal, healthy, young men who drank ice-cold drinks after playing football and had heart attacks. Dr. Lamb says the reasons are not entirely clear, but apparently cold may bring on a coronary artery spasm and obstruct the blood supply to the heart muscle.

There is often a tendency to let the first water break come too late in the practice or competitive event. Even the International Amateur Athletic Federation fell into this trap when they ruled that there had to be water stops every 3 miles in the 26.2 mile marathon races, *but only after the first 7*. On a hot day, some of the runners' fluid and electrolyte loss in those 7 miles is irreversible during the race. Replacement can only occur from nutrition and rest afterwards. However, the amount that is irreversible can be minimized by prehydration and much earlier fluid and electrolyte replacement in any athletic event; but if any of the symptoms of heat illness develop, the athlete should stop immediately and the coach must use his judgment as to whether a medical referral is advisable. It is strongly recommended that he err on the conservative side.

News articles on the Boston Marathon often mention the number of runners who are laid out on stretchers after the race and that, on occasion, doctors even administer oxygen. In addition, you will frequently hear runners talk about their dehydration and muscle spasms after the race. In most cases these symptoms can be alleviated, or prevented, by more hydration with proper electrolyte fluids during the race, and immediate hydration at the finish line. Since reporters insist on hounding these good runners, the least race officials can do is to have someone there who will shove a big paper cup of an electrolyte fluid into the runner's hand, which he can sip while talking to the reporters.

Individual Tolerances

The decision to administer an electrolyte solution during exercise must be made by the coach or individual athlete based on his ability to tolerate it. If his stomach won't accept it during the event, he has to make it up in electrolyte fluids before and afterward, or at meals. In any case, for the athlete with a tolerance problem, a more dilute solution or plain water should be available. Regardless of which fluid is used, he must be trained to drink a quantity as near to 90 percent of total replacement as he can without feeling so full that it affects his performance adversely.

There was a practical example of the difference in individual tolerance, in this case in relation to salt, in Colin

Fletcher's *The Complete Walker*. Fletcher undertook to walk alone through Death Valley, where he encountered daytime ground temperatures of up to 120° F. After a few hairy incidents, he succeeded, and in his comments about salt said: "Individual requirements vary widely. A Death Valley ranger once told me, 'When it reaches 110° F. I take one tablet a day. I need more, but my stomach won't accept more. Yet there's a guy at Park HQ who has to take twenty a day. If he doesn't he ends up in the hospital.'"

As in the Death Valley ranger's story, individual requirements and tolerances vary widely due to differences in hormonal response. Furthermore, there is strong evidence that well-conditioned individuals, who will be almost fully acclimatized to heat in about a week, can hang on to both sodium chloride and potassium better than untrained individuals, who retain sodium chloride at the expense of potassium. For the conditioned individuals the addition of electrolytes to fluid may be reduced, depending on heat and weather conditions, and the potential potassium deficit can usually be avoided by eating a potassium-rich diet. (Potassium-rich foods may be found in *Composition of Foods—Raw, Processed, Prepared*, Agriculture Handbook No. 8.) However, the relative proportion of electrolytes in fluids is going to be up to the medical advisor and the coach, who may elect to use periodic blood testing as the most accurate method of determining the condition and the need of each athlete. On a more frequent basis a simple urine test can now be done, which will indicate the sodium chloride content and thus any grossly abnormal situations can be picked up. This test is done by means of a small chemical device, graduated like a thermometer, which is placed in the urine the day after a strenuous event. Known as Quantab, it is manufactured by Ames Company, Division of Miles Laboratory, Inc., Elkhart, Indiana, and is simpler to perform than the traditional Fantus test, which is done by silver nitrate titration.

A problem with stomach irritation can be avoided by eliminating the use of salt tablets. During stressful competition, undissolved tablets can be harmful as they draw fluids back into the gut for dilution purposes, and in some individuals can cause discomfort and even incapacitation. Consequently, salt tablets taken indiscriminately without sufficient water can compound the whole heat and weight loss problem.

We do not know of any large sample studies of runners that indicate no electrolytes at all are needed, although there may be individual runners in superb physical condition who can and do function without them. Again, it is debatable whether they might not perform even better with carefully controlled ingestion of electrolytes in solution. However, the weight of evidence indicates that in any high-stress exercise where there is substantial weight loss, heat, a long period of time involved, or all three, not any one electrolyte alone but a variety of dissolved electrolytes should be taken, subject to individual tolerance, in solutions no stronger than those mentioned below.

Medical and Scientific Theories

The old myth that an athlete shouldn't take fluids during high-stress exercise came from the fact that if he drinks large amounts of water without electrolytes, it can dilute the concentration of the body fluids so much that he will get muscle cramps. This prompted the theory that the water caused the cramps, rather than the lack of electrolytes, in this case specifically salt.

In the early '30s Dr. Dill advised a steel company to put .1 percent salt in solution (1 gram or 15 grains per quart) in all the water available to blast-furnace operators, who at first refused to drink it. When they finally tried it and found that cramps and other illnesses disappeared, all the men in the plant wanted it.

Currently Dr. Richard L. Westerman, Senior Clinical Research Physician, Upjohn International, recommends this same amount of salt, plus 750–950 mg. of potassium added to the solution. The potassium is the equivalent of one dissolved tablet, trademarked as K-Lyte, per liter.

Rather than mix one's own salt and potassium, Dr. Westerman suggests two or three commercial premixed powders (see pages 207–210) that contain additional electrolytes. These preparations must be mixed accurately, as excessively strong solutions cause problems by temporarily drawing water out of the body into the gut for dilution purposes, thus defeating the purpose of the fluid. With a properly diluted mixture, he recommends that one pint of the electrolyte fluid be drunk per pound of weight loss, up to 90 percent of replacement, based on an advance estimate and within known tolerance limits.

But if the athlete drinks too much he will go beyond his comfort limit and impair his performance. This limit can only be determined by experience, as it depends to some extent on his rate of gastric emptying, which varies from 1 to 1⅔ pints of fluid per hour. Most people can drink 6–8 ounces every 15 minutes.

Another authority on use of fluids in high-stress exercise, Dr. David L. Costill of Ball State University, has reported on distance running, saying that water and salt loss in sweat and decreased muscle sugar are major factors in fatigue during severe, long-duration exercise. If sweat is replaced with salt and water, and glucose supplied, the athlete's performance should be improved. Strenuous exercise does not seriously affect absorption by the small intestine and any minor slowing in the rate of stomach emptying can be largely offset by drinking water with .1 percent salt solution and 5 percent or less glucose. Stronger glucose and salt mixtures (hypertonic) slow down the emptying process, and, even with the optimum solution, glucose has a limited rate of absorption, which can only replace 25–50 percent of the amount of body fuel expended.

On a hot day the circulatory system has a doubly hard job, both feeding muscles and getting rid of excess heat through the skin. High humidity compounds this, since the sweat does not evaporate as fast and its cooling effect is minimized. Particularly with a bright sun, the skin should be covered with light, loose, white clothing, to reflect the radiance of the sun. Dr. Costill says: "The acute dehydration that accompanies profuse sweating while running in the heat causes a reduction in extracellular fluid and a significant lowering of the runner's blood volume." Like a half-filled car radiator in summer, the body overheats and the heart has to pump harder to get its job done.

Body temperatures of 104–106° F. have been recorded among marathon runners in the heat, which can only be tolerated by the superbly conditioned. An unfit person would be in serious trouble with heat exhaustion or heat stroke long before he reached those temperatures. Great care must be taken by both coaches and athletes that no one go beyond his level of acclimatization and physical condition.

Dr. Gerard Balakian, practicing internist in New Jersey, an experienced advisor to team physicians, and Fellow of the American College of Clinical Pharmacology, recommends not only salt and potassium, but also a spectrum of electrolytes in correct proportions. These include: sodium, potassium, chloride, and carbohydrates in a palatable, nonirritating drink. This should be taken continuously during exercise in 6–8-ounce portions. The total consumed should be governed by 85–90 percent of weight lost previously under like conditions of temperature, humidity, type of exercise, and clothing worn.

Dr. Balakian has developed a formula for an electrolyte solution, which has worked successfully with numerous athletic teams that have tested it. It contains the equivalent per quart of 1.25 grams of salt, 675 mg. of potassium, plus calcium, magnesium, Vitamin C, and a quickly available carbohydrate.

Sea Salt

Body fluids lost through sweat come principally from fluid outside the body's cells (extracellular fluid). Movement from one compartment to another occurs by filtration through a membrane, but even so, the hormonal system and the kidneys do a marvelous and intricate job in keeping these compartments in balance through the homeostatic mechanism.

The composition of the extracellular fluid, which is lost in exercise, has been compared many times to sea water, which it somewhat resembles. The suggestion has been advanced that, at one time, before membranes created the walls of the compartments, water from the seas flowed in and out as our tiny cellular ancestors squirmed and wiggled in the Precambrian oceans. However, in the aeons since these membranes came into being, the seas have increased enormously in salinity due to leaching and evaporation, so the resemblance has diminished as geologic time has passed.

We have used sea salt in distance running, in proper amounts, instead of table salt. Sea salt means the salts and minerals of the first evaporation of sea water. (Unfortunately, a number of products on the market labeled "Sea Salt" have been so refined from the original ocean salt that they are no more than ordinary table salt, at four times the supermarket price.) It contains about 77 percent of the sodium chloride of ordinary salt, plus magnesium, calcium, and phosphate, but not enough potassium to reach recommended levels. In addition it probably contains enough trace minerals to answer requirements for those elements. Our impression is that it is not as irritating as plain salt, and seems to work well enough even though it's a crude imitation of the extracellular spectrum of electrolytes.

In weak (.1 percent) hypotonic solutions it seems harmless, even though a bit high in sulfates, which would only have a laxative effect in a large quantity. Otherwise, we would have heard adversely from people who live along the shore and consume large quantities of clams, oysters, and other marine shellfish that contain considerable amounts of sea salt.

Aerobics author, Dr. Kenneth H. Cooper, did a study of marathon runners, in which he found that over a period of time, particularly in warm weather, they tend to show a loss of magnesium from both the blood serum and the cellular tissue. He recommends that runners take two dolomite tablets at each meal. This gives a total of approximately 780 mg. of calcium and 468 mg. of magnesium per day, which Dr. Cooper considers to be in the right proportion as well as an adequate amount of these two important electrolytes.

Dolomite is a natural and inexpensive source of calcium and magnesium. (Where used in this book, "natural" means "as it occurs in nature"—unprocessed and unpreserved by any method, with nothing added and nothing taken away, except impurities not related to or part of the item itself.) In addition, orange juice is a good natural source of potassium. It contains 1,041 mg. per pint of fresh juice and 968 mg. per pint of reconstituted juice. For those athletes who like to make their own concoctions, a mixture of half orange juice and half water with 1 gram of sea salt dissolved per quart makes a palatable and nonirritating electrolyte drink with about 234 calories per quart of easily digested carbohydrates. (Get your druggist to show you how to measure 1 gram.) Then take the dolomite regularly and you are well protected with a balance of electrolytes. Some runners even take the dolomite before and during workouts and competition.

Another concoction can be made by dissolving 2 ounces (by weight) of blackstrap molasses in one quart of water. Add 1 gram of sea salt and this quart will provide, in addition to the salt, 400 mg. of calcium, 184 mg. of magnesium, 1,671 mg. of potassium, and 121 calories of carbohydrates. The only problem may be tolerating the molasses flavor. If you're one of those who can't, try the orange juice mixture or one of the commercial preparations.

Other Points of View

There is another point of view, which does not agree with the use of electrolytes and advocates full fluid replacement only with plain water. Dr. Laurence M. Hursch, Head of the Division of Environmental Health, University of Illinois, takes this position based on U.S. Army studies for men walking up a 2½ percent grade at 3.5 mph for a period of hours.

While we suggest that this could only be called high-stress output in terms of its very long duration, there are definite reasons why the Army and also many doctors disapprove of the use of too much salt, principally because excessive use of salt has been implicated in high blood pressure. Furthermore, many trainers and athletes are beginning to question its use in high-stress athletics and because the amount needed varies widely according to individual tolerances. In addition, Dr. Hursch objects to the use of salt because it is frequently taken in tablet form, causing irritation and gastric upset.

The Army position against salt is supported by Dr. David E. Bass of the U.S. Army Research Institute of Environmental Medicine, who, in addition, does not feel that potassium need be added to fluids and that it should be replaced nutritionally.

In a paper published in the *South African Medical Journal,* Drs. C. H. Wyndham and N. B. Strydom cover very thoroughly the need for adequate fluid (water) in marathon running. However, since no mention is made of electrolytes in any form, it may be assumed that they do not regard them as important or necessary.

From a totally different source comes another objection to salt from champion distance runner Dr. (Ph.D. in Mathematics) Tom Osler, who has set National AAU records for 25 and 30 kilometers. He has not said much about it except that he trains and races without it and maintains that as a result he is better off.

Summary

When presented with conflicting opinions, one must study the background, the research, and reports of practical application. After weighing all aspects, we have based the following conclusions on the preponderance of the evidence:

1. Whereas plain water is better than no fluid at all, it can cause problems when taken alone in large amounts over long periods.

2. Salt without sufficient water can be irritating and even dangerous.

3. Salt and water in the right proportions are helpful, but can stimulate a loss of potassium, calcium, and magnesium, which suggests that those who advise against it may really mean no salt without the other electrolytes.

4. The need for potassium has been demonstrated by Dr. Gerard Balakian and others.

5. The need for calcium and magnesium has been demonstrated with respect to distance runners by Dr. Kenneth H. Cooper. Therefore, the logical conclusion seems to be for the athlete to drink a solution of the proper strength containing a balanced spectrum of the electrolytes of the body fluids so that those that are lost in sweating can be anticipated and replaced.

Weight losses must be estimated in advance from training experience, making due allowance for heat (or cold), clothing worn, and humidity; when the estimate is made, fluids must be taken before, during, and after to 85–90 percent of replacement. It is important that this program be developed in training so it can be followed automatically in competition, with full cooperation between the coach or trainer and the athlete.

Given these general guidelines, the following lists the ingredients in some of the electrolyte products that are available commercially and also the two homemade mixtures:

ELECTROLYTE PREPARATIONS

Commercial Name	Mfrs. Unit	Ingredients	Amount per Unit	Amount per Quart
BRAKE TIME	1 packet	Calories	128	32
(Available through	added to	Sodium	1,792 mg.	448 mg.
athletic distributors	1 Gal.	Potassium	1,408 mg.	352 mg.
or directly from	water	Sodium		
Johnson & Johnson		Saccharin	768 mg.	192 mg.
Athletic Division,		Vitamin C	213 mg.	53 mg.
New Brunswick,				
New Jersey 08903)				

Ingredients: Glucose, sucrose, citric acid, monobasic potassium phosphate, salt, sodium citrate, artificial and natural flavors, potassium chloride, sodium saccharin, Vitamin C, and artificial color.

One of the more recent electrolyte drinks to come on the market, BRAKE TIME, has reduced carbohydrate content in line with the theory that without it the body learns to burn its own fat when stored glycogen runs low. In addition, medical and scientific authorities have begun to frown on heavy intake of refined carbohydrates during exercise on the basis that after an initial lift, there is a letdown due to functional hypoglycemia.

Commercial Name	Mfrs. Unit	Ingredients	Amount per Unit	Amount per Quart
SIDE-LINE SIDER	1 packet	Calories	831	208
(Available from	added to	Sodium	2,202 mg.	551 mg.
Cramer Products, Inc.,	1 Gal.	Chloride	3,398 mg.	849 mg.
Gardner, Kansas	water	Potassium	2,665 mg.	666 mg.
66030)		Citrate	4,335 mg.	1,084 mg.

Ingredients: Sugar, glucose, fumaric acid, citric acid, sodium chloride, potassium citrate, artificial flavors and coloring, and sodium benzoate (preservative).

Contains sufficient sodium, chloride, and potassium. It is a well-balanced solution of the three major electrolytes.

Commercial Name	Mfrs. Unit	Item	Amount per Unit	Amount per Quart
E.R.G.	1 packet added to 1 Gal. water	(This information is not made available. However, the formula for E.R.G. was developed by trained chemist and marathoner Bill Gookin of San Diego. It is based on an analysis of his sweat. "The Runner's Diet," published by *Runner's World* magazine reports that it contains balanced proportions of sodium and potassium, Vitamin C, and buffers for maintaining acid-alkaline balance.)		

Ingredients: Glucose, citric acid, sodium chloride, potassium chloride, ascorbic acid (Vitamin C), sodium bicarbonate, dibasic potassium phosphate, magnesium and calcium carbonates, natural citrus flavor, and U.S. certified color.

	Item	Amount per Quart
ORANGE JUICE MIXTURE (RECONSTITUTED)	Calories	234
	Sodium	311 mg.
	Chloride	553 mg.
	Potassium	979 mg.
Ingredients: Orange juice, sea salt (See recipe on page 204)	Phosphorous	83 mg.
	Magnesium	90 mg.
	Calcium	59 mg.
	Plus Trace of Minerals	

	Item	Amount per Quart
BLACK STRAP MOLASSES MIXTURE	Calories	121
	Sodium	360 mg.
	Chloride	553 mg.
	Potassium	1,671 mg.
	Phosphorous	48 mg.
Ingredients: Black strap	Calcium	400 mg.
molasses, sea salt (See	Magnesium	184 mg.
recipe on page 204)	Plus Trace of Minerals	

Commercial Name	Mfrs. Unit	Item	Amount per Unit	Amount per Quart
GATORADE	32 oz.	Calories	160	160
(Available from super-		Sodium	512 mg.	512 mg.
markets or directly from		Potassium	96 mg.	96 mg.
Stokely-Van Camp, In-		Saccharin	67 mg.	67 mg.
dianapolis, Indiana, in				
powder or bottled form.				
Originally developed at				
the University of				
Florida)				

Ingredients: Water, glucose, fructose, citric acid, salt, sodium citrate, sodium orthophosphate, potassium orthophosphate, potassium chloride, natural and artificial flavors, ester gum, sodium saccharin and artificial color.

Contains insufficient potassium.

This whole subject of fluid and electrolyte management in high-stress exercise needs further research with group and individual testing. To date, our knowledge of it is undoubtedly less than the tip of the iceberg. In any event, from the currently available evidence and weight of

opinion, the above preparations are similar to the electrolyte spectrum of body fluids, and therefore appropriate for
replacement in this order:

BRAKE TIME (the best from a formula and flavor standpoint).

SIDE-LINE SIDER

E.R.G. (This is a pleasant and palatable drink; however, the mystery about its ingredients puts it at a disadvantage).

As alternatives, try the homemade mixtures. They have
plenty of potassium and neither of them has any of the refined sugars, which is a serious disadvantage with all the
commercial preparations except Brake Time.

A choice of an electrolyte drink should be made to be
used in training and competition and a program followed.
From there on, let the hormones and the kidneys make
their homeostatic selections from the fluids and the foods
that we put before them.

12 The Relationship Between Physical and Mental Health

"Wherever there is a heart and an intellect, the diseases of the physical frame are tinged with the peculiarities of these."
Nathaniel Hawthorne:
The Scarlet Letter

Like the St. John River in Canada, this relationship flows in both directions because, as Hawthorne suggested, physical condition can influence mental attitude and, conversely, mental health or illness can affect the individual physically. This does not imply that if an individual is seriously disturbed strenuous physical activity will cure him, because obviously he needs medical assistance. But for everyday stresses and problems, strength and cardiopulmonary fitness will help by providing a healthy autonomic (involuntary) nervous system as a background on which to resolve them. This stability is achieved when exercise burns up the products of physical response to emotional stress in the "fight or flight" adrenaline cycle.

This whole bidirectional relationship was expressed so well by the late President John F. Kennedy: "But we do know what the Greeks knew: That intelligence and skill can only function at the peak of their capacity when the body is healthy and strong; that hardy spirits and tough minds usually inhabit sound bodies."

The first part of the late president's thesis is especially relevant here. Although keen intelligence is largely hereditary, skill must be developed. But both the inherited intelligence and the developed skill need a proper climate in which to function at their peak. Therefore, maximum mental skill and achievement can best be attained along with an active and healthful physical life. Conversely, the unhealthy, unconditioned college professor, doctor, lawyer, or businessman will probably not work at his peak efficiency if he is in a poor fitness category due to bad diet, lack of exercise, and heavy smoking or drinking.

The need to avoid these exposures was emphasized in the past by studies of pilots and aircrews, who must maintain a high degree of physical fitness. While the decisions and actions of airmen are classically critical in nature, the earth-bound professional or businessman can still cause a lot of grief for himself and others from deteriorated judgment or presence of mind.

A loss of efficiency can be caused by business upsets, family problems, or money worries, or by organic reasons, which must be treated by a doctor. So if a medical examination reveals no organic illness, a magnification of the problem is probably caused by psychic tensions, in which case exercise should help. These tensions frequently bring about physiological changes that result in disfunction, discomfort, or illness. As any physician knows, they cause more problems today in medicine than infectious diseases. The causal relationship between emotional tension and physical disturbances was originally explicated by Harvard physiologist Walter B. Cannon in his *Bodily Changes in Pain, Hunger, Fear and Rage,* a work that has influenced the field of psychophysiologic medicine.

Chronic emotional stress will usually strike the weakest or most susceptible part of the body in the form of discomfort, sometimes without demonstrable organic cause. When a part of the body breaks down this way under such stress, it is known as "somatic compliance." In many such cases treatment by a specialist who understands therapeutic exercise may bring long- or short-term relief. Obviously, the best course is to eliminate the cause. But if this can't be done, the sufferer has to learn to live with the problem and a well-planned course of exercise with strong aerobic emphasis will be of tremendous benefit.

Although the following example has a different technical pattern, it is a good illustration of how a specific problem can arise and is then treated. A woman developed a severe back pain every time she planned to take a trip by air. The stress and tension from her deep-seated fear of flying caused excessive glandular activity two or three days before the proposed trip. The focal point, or point of somatic compliance, of the stress was her back, which became extremely painful. Her fear of flying was the primary cause of the physiologic response of the back pain. In a limited sense, this is known as a conversion reaction, which met her immediate need of not having to fly. Her ultimate need of being able to fly calmly and without pain was met by a program of regular exercise. This was nature's own tranquilizer, so that after several months on the program the pain did not recur, even when a trip by air was planned.

Like all one-man statistics, there is no proof that the exercise was the cause of the relief. However, it did at least improve the woman's outlook and sense of well-being to the extent that she was able to relax and approach a flight with a more reasonable perspective. This in itself undoubtedly helped to modify the emotional disturbance with its resultant physiological reaction.

Since the era of President Kennedy, there has been a revolution in our concept of ourselves and our society. The counterculture of the 1970s has pointed out vociferously, and with much justification, that there is a monumental array of bad, dishonest, unattractive, and dangerous things in our world today, made more objectionable by the perversion of our attitudes and life styles with a Madison Avenue type of dishonesty and hypocrisy. An example is the business executive who drinks martinis at lunch, takes sleeping pills at night, and while still under the influence of either or both declaims loudly against pot. This conflict is age-old and is beautifully illustrated by Mark Twain in *Huckleberry Finn,* when he tells about his difficulties in staying with the widow.

"Pretty soon I wanted to smoke, and asked the widow to let me. But she wouldn't. She said it was a mean practice and wasn't clean, and I must try to not do it any more. That is just the way with some people. . . . And she took snuff, too; of course that was all right, because she done it herself."

From any point of view, we would be far better off without all these drugs, which are insidious and vicious mistreaters of the human body. Because of the profound relationship between mind and body, this physical mistreatment, which at the start is entirely avoidable, affects mental health and attitude.

Only rare individuals can overcome the effect upon the mind of poor health, from whatever cause. An extreme example of mistreatment of the human body occurs in malnutrition and semistarvation, which adversely affect both mental capacity and frame of reference. In prisoners of war, one of us (JSF) observed that as food intake drops, points of view change; very gradually at first, and then as diet deteriorates well below the subsistence level, the prisoner becomes a different person, and eventually takes some of the attitudes toward food that are associated with aggressive animals.

Captured in North Africa, JSF was sent with a group of American prisoners to a barbed-wire transient camp near Capua in Italy, where they were confined to a separate quadrangle. Occasionally, their captors would assign them the task of going to a commissary in another part of the compound to bring back baskets of the meager rations that provided a plate of soup and a small roll twice a day, supplemented by an occasional orange. Since Red Cross parcels had not reached the camp, several weeks of this had introduced them to degrees of hunger that they were scarcely equipped to handle. The effect of their relationship with each other was tension, irritability, and moodiness. On one occasion JSF was given the detail, along with two other prisoners, of picking up a couple of baskets of oranges from the commissary. On the way back they had to pass through an area occupied by some British prisoners, who had been captured a year and a half before. Some of them had been kept in cages and by contrast the Americans, who thought they were hungry, were fat cats, while the scrawny necks of the British stuck out of their shirt collars like pipe stems. Out of sunken eyes they glared with savage hostility at the men with the oranges. Suddenly, there was a stir and one of them grabbed at the nearest basket. He was blocked off and the detail marched on, but two or three oranges rolled on the ground. Despite shouted orders from the guards, the group of prisoners broke and scrambled for those oranges like wild dogs after a piece of meat. During the scuffle, the guard whisked the detail through a gate and returned them to their hut, shaken by what they had seen.

The British prisoners were from highly disciplined units, but they had had such a bad time that they had lost their frame of reference. Capua was a temporary stop and undoubtedly the overcrowded conditions and forced inactivity had added to the problem. However, several months later, along with some men who had been through a similar experience, the Americans were sent to a permanent camp where there was more room for activity. A few of these men were great walkers, and by striding round and round the camp in areas where they were permitted to do so, they regained a reasonable degree of normality and were able to adjust to the confinement.

JSF and another American prisoner started some calisthenics classes. Through these it was clearly demonstrated that prisoners who forced themselves, in spite of their hunger, to be active physically and mentally had greater ability to resist the deterioration caused by hunger and confinement. This was in spite of dire predictions and sometimes severe criticism on the part of fellow prisoners. The contrast between the British and Americans was great. The British were more oriented toward fitness, while few Americans seemed to be aware of the absolute necessity to maintain activity as a requisite to physical and mental survival.

The prisoner-of-war case is an example of how Americans tend to ignore this psychophysical relationship, and continue to do so to a greater extent today. Beyond ignoring, there have even been at some universities rhetorical attacks on athletes, as if they were some type of sinister influence in the academic community.

Contrary to American attitudes, Soviet studies of planned, regular physical activity in relation to on-the-job efficiency and sound mental attitude are some of the finest ever done. The Soviets recognize strongly the importance and depth of this relationship and we can take a lesson from them.

There has been a great deal written in recent years about the meaninglessness of American life. This lack of belonging, of roots or identity, afflicts younger people and those in business somewhat more frequently than those in the professions, arts, and sciences. But there is a later time in life when we are particularly susceptible to it. This has been recognized by writers and philosophers for centuries and Dante deemed it important enough to start the first canto of the "Inferno" with this thought:

> Midway upon the journey of our life
> I found myself within a forest dark,
> For the straightforward pathway had been lost.

For hundreds of years since Dante, this mood and feeling of middle life was thought of in spiritual or psychic terms. Only recently has it been given a biochemical explanation. This was done magnificently by Cameron Hawley in *The Hurricane Years*, where Dr. Aaron Kharr is describing to his postcoronary patient, Judd Wilder, what has happened to him:

> However, as he comes into middle age, typically in his mid-forties, adequate stimulation becomes difficult to find. The old challenges have lost their potency. There are few situations that he has not faced before, few problems for which his experience will not quickly supply an answer. The hope for further advancement has often dimmed. His personal life has commonly become routine, equally lacking in future promise. For most men, this is a period of crisis. A few respond by radically reordering their lives, changing jobs or even entering some entirely new field, but it is only the exceptional man to whom that opportunity is available. Most men, surely the majority, settle back and adjust to a lower level of adrenaline stimulation. But not the man we are examining. He has, in the idiom of the drug addict, become so hooked on adrenaline that he can't kick the habit. Unable to find sufficiently stimulating major challenges, he begins to rely on a multiplicity of minor ones. When they do not exist, he invents them. Quite unknowingly, he starts playing little adrenal-stimulating games. One of the most commonly observed is a running battle with the clock and the calendar. By constantly fighting the pressure of time, he can generate a continuing air of crisis, and thus keep giving himself repeated shots of adrenaline all day long.

Dr. Kharr has explained to his patient how the adrenal glands make adrenaline, or more accurately, norepinephrine, as a response to psychic challenge. While they are doing that, the rest of the body seems to be unable to make a critical polysaccharide called heparin, which is needed to clear the blood of undesirable fat cells that are chemically bound to glycerine as triglycerides. If the fat is not removed, these triglycerides thicken the blood until it becomes like sludge. Now the man is in constant danger of a heart attack from a blockage in a narrowed coronary artery.

Admittedly, the reversal of this person's way of life must be both prompt and dramatic in order to avoid catastrophe, but it is by no means impossible. His whole existence can be brought into sharp, meaningful focus by the right kind of stimulation of his adrenal glands, the kind that will allow the resumption of a balanced output of nor-epinephrine and heparin. The malaise and the feeling of having lost his way will disappear and he will gradually acquire immeasurably greater ability to withstand the stresses of life and he will regain his sense of direction.

This principle applies even for those in reduced economic circumstances where diet is marginal. The benefit of physical activity was shown by the prisoner-of-war example, which clearly demonstrated that, although on the most deficient and minimal diet, the active men were more alert, felt better, and were more able to cope with the difficulties of the situation than the completely inactive and sedentary ones.

Almost every aspect of our environment today creates some kind of stress that emphasizes our need for ways to counteract it. We can do the obvious things that must be done to ensure our survival: get rid of air pollution, eliminate crowded city areas and the illnesses that go with them, and cut out the horrible waste in the United States. (Due to overportioning and lack of concern, enough valuable food to bring subsistence to millions of underfed Americans ends up in garbage pails. In fact in a tragic way, it does bring subsistence to some. Young people who run away from home often manage to live out of the garbage cans of the same kind of troubled families they have left.)

Above all things, we must learn what to eat and how and where to obtain it, and that physical activity is an absolute necessity as a part of our way of life. Then we shall all be better equipped to adjust to the rapidly accelerating technology.

As we stand in the midst of this technological torrent, compounding its speed at an ever-increasing rate, we watch and wonder what will happen to the human personality, a product of hundreds and thousands of years of mammalian heredity, which is totally unsuited to this rate of change.

Alvin Toffler, in *Future Shock,* quoted Julian Huxley as saying that "The tempo of human evolution during recorded history is at least 100,000 times as rapid as that of pre-human evolution." No doubt biologist Huxley knew what he was talking about, but Mr. Toffler leaves the impression that human evolution is currently taking on an increased tempo, which, if true, might offer a partial solution. However, we see no evidence that human evolutionary changes are keeping pace with technology. Quite to the contrary, the gap in our ability to adjust only seems to widen, leaving the majority, who try to keep up, stumbling neurotically behind, unhappy victims of a system and an environment to which they are unable to adapt. Those few do better who do not try to adapt, but instead strike off in other directions, toward higher and more enlightened levels of consciousness, states which by their very nature reject technology and its materialism.

If this gap between the evolutionary change and the technological rate of change continues to widen, human adaptation must at some point fall behind to the extent where it can no longer relate. The geneticists and molecular biologists may think they can play Pygmalion with our adaptive responses, but they all could end up as Dr. Frankensteins with some unpredictable imbalance of nature.

To maintain a sense of balance between our evolutionary capabilities and our changing environment we shall need mental, physical, and spiritual strength. Since scientific knowledge is probably accumulating faster than our ability to handle it, offered here is a method to fortify ourselves against these stresses, a method that can bring with it a sense of well-being and happiness so that maybe, in this turbulent world in which we live, we can keep our perspective and even devote a little time to the joy of living.

13 An Impossible Dream (JSF Runs the Boston Marathon)

While life has an ebb and flow to it, there are plateaus in between on which we stay, sometimes for a long time. But many of us become restless when we are caught on a plateau because we are attuned to the rhythmic cycles of life—day and night, sleep and action, winter and summer—and thus from time to time we like a change.

So if you've enjoyed the upper realms of this experience for a while and you begin to fret and want to reach for distant stars, here is a look at the road ahead.

It came to me as a canter along the aisle of fantasy early one spring morning. The air was very cool and still. Green buds were on the branches of the maples and the woods rang with bird song. As I ran along that morning, I lengthened my stride and felt as if I could run forever. With the euphoria of good health and a bit of spring madness it hit me! Why not train for the Boston Marathon? I was both excited and appalled by the idea, but not as appalled as I would have been if I had only known.

Hal Hidgon, in his witty and entertaining book, *On the Run from Dogs and People,* finishes with some pretty professional comments on marathon racing. Far be it from me to venture into the rarified atmosphere of his world of great runners. My peer group is composed of fellow fugitives from tobacco, alcohol, and cholesterol, who are graciously allowed to run, I mean jog, in nearly all the club and open races and championships, which recognize age groups up to 70 years old.

But my glimpse of the stars came long after that summer and fall when my fantasy first began to take hold. Having done no more than 3 or 4 miles at a time, I added 2 miles each month to the length of my runs—too much mileage too quickly—and soon I began to go very slowly. But, without realizing it, I was building a cardiopulmonary base and strengthening muscles, tendons, and ligaments without the danger of injury from fast work. I applied for Boston before the days of the 3½-hour requirement and got my number. (In late 1970, Boston marathon officials, overwhelmed with entrants and problems they create on a straight-away course from Hopkinton into Boston's heaviest traffic, ruled out the enthusiastic joggers and restricted their race to the elite by accepting no entrant unless he had previously completed an alternate of certain qualification times, the principal one of which was an official AAU marathon in under 3½ hours.)

Every Boston Marathon has a thousand stories, some

painful, some tragic, and some ecstatic. Besides the brilliant, fabulously trained runner who gets the laurel wreath, there are hundreds of others who win their own private battles.

This race is held on Patriot's Day, which now is a Monday late in April. So throughout March I pushed hard, doing alternately 75 and 90 miles a week, and began to border on exhaustion. With 4½ hours sleep some nights, I never quite caught up. I had originally worked out a schedule of rounding-out exercises, which I later modified, and my nagging aches and pains were greatly alleviated by a lightened program including flexibility and stretching.

On Friday, April 17, a beautiful warm day, I left home in the station wagon and headed for Cambridge, loaded with Gatorade, clothes for all weather, and a splitting headache that got worse as I went north. I thought of a virus and Asiatic flu, but it was pure tension and I finally made it to Cambridge, where I spent the night.

The next morning my friend, Bill Barry, a physician and great athlete, drove me to the start of the marathon in Hopkinton. With Bill exuding enthusiasm, we made a plan for the race, so by the time my wife Emmie arrived that evening my confidence had begun to return. Maybe my crazy idea was possible after all.

Monday, April 20, 3:15 A.M., 26.21875 miles to go and all I can think of is where's the next toilet. My shoes are lost and I have to run in a brand new pair, never worn; visions of blisters as big as poached eggs.

At 7:00 A.M. I have an enormous bowl of porridge and whole wheat bread. It's 48° and a cold rain. Resting pulse rate up from 60 to 72. Emmie and I drive to Hopkinton in the wagon. Tacitly, she is horrified at how far it is. The town is still empty and as we park the car it's getting colder by the minute. We go to the wrong school to sign in and be examined. I get sent away to the high school down Hayward Row. The big, lofty gym is crowded with long lines of men getting their numbers. They are outwardly calm and murmuring, but there is high tension in the air. All sizes, shapes, ages, and talents; a dozen or so men my age; but a sense of fundamental equality in what we confront together; each individual in those last miles must face himself.

There is a lump in my throat and an awesome hollow in my stomach. My hands fumble nervously with my card and drop it on the floor. Before I can bend over, a runner who could be my grandson swoops it up and hands it to me with an embarrassed smile.

I stand in the wrong line for a while, then recognize a friendly voice shouting, "Hey, Joe, over here." It's Dr. Warren Guild, my coach and enthusiastic sponsor, who has my record. He has run the Boston Marathon many times, once in two hours, fifty-six minutes. As he stamps my card, his smiling wink and the warmth of his handshake give me a momentary reprieve from the death-cell quality of my mood.

I get my number, 437, and we drive back to the starting line, where we meet my daughter, Susan. The temperature is 43° and it's still raining. I get more chilled and try to warm up, putting on more clothes and leaving my gloves—both errors.

Ron Hill is the favorite as the greatest marathoners in the world line up in front on Hayward Row. I'm back 40 feet behind the line, where the runners are genially kidding each other. There are Saran-wrap hats and gloves, shivering men in sleeveless shirts, and tiny track pants. I have sweater and jacket, and long pants.

Noon. The gun goes "pop," while television cameras grind and the leaders burst off like sprinters, Drayton and Hill in the lead. Back where I am, the mob surges and telescopes.

"Hey, move out, you guys!"

"Get going up there."

Like a bobbing river of red, orange, white, green, and blue the men flow ahead filling the road. Strong and husky runners are followed by the odds and ends, the flotsam and jetsam of this great race. They are the soft and untrained, who can never finish. They are the serious, gray-haired men, with drawn, lined faces, who will, or will not, this day defy once more time's immutable and inescapable destiny.

They stretch out down the long, curving hill of Route 135 and up the rise toward Ashland. Far ahead the champion runners have blasted into the lead with mile after mile at five minutes and under, in a drenching downpour through the shopping centers of Framingham, the spired red brick New England town of Natick, and the chic opulence of Wellesley Hills.

Ron Hill is in the lead, in violent rhythm, 192 strides to the minute; he is averaging 4:59 per mile in rain spattering on the macadam. Orange-slickered police stand motionless at the crossings, holding the vibrating traffic in check, and the umbrella-packed crowd cheers Hill on as he tears toward an all-time record.

Back in Ashland, the open press trucks come up along side me, honking, all pointed cameras and up-turned hat brims. I'm overwhelmed with delight, until I realize there are some women running behind me and the photographers are taking their pictures.

It's pouring. My feet squish in cold puddles and, picking up water, my clothes are heavy and dank. My legs are stiff and my throat feels sore. A man of about 60, in a green toque and shirt, pads resolutely by me. I can tell by his stride that he knows his business. There is another man about my age, apparently crippled with arthritis, running with a long-legged shuffle. I pass him coming into Framingham, then he passes when I stop for a drink at the car, though I'm out in less than a minute. Beyond Framingham, up the grade at barely mile 9, I begin to feel the drag. My leg aches from the wet and cold. It feels like a charley horse; I see myself rolling on the wet pavement in a spasm. The going is flat, but I feel myself slowing. It pours again and my clothes pick up more water, and my shoes splash in the running water.

At Wellesley College the action has passed and the girls are gone. One hoots at me from the top floor, kidding the tardy plodder. In town, the streets are deserted and more orange-coated police are still holding traffic. I slog down the middle of the empty wide street in the pouring rain, where I come upon a man in a wheelchair, pumping along in the middle of the road. There are quotes from the Bible on his chair. As I go by and say "hello," he answers in a keyed-up voice: "Believe in Jesus, brother, and be saved." I mumble awkwardly and keep going, and hear him singing a hymn in a strong clear voice. He is Eugene Roberts from Baltimore. He started at eleven and would finish at six, a former runner who lost both legs in Vietnam.

On Route 16, in heavy traffic, a horn blasts a few feet behind me and a "lady" in a Cadillac pulls by, shaking her fist; I'm with the kids against the Establishment.

I overtake a heavy young man, 20 or so, walking. He picks up a jog alongside me and wants to know how much farther it is. I say 10; but it's 12. I'm slowing as we reach

Newton Lower Falls. I grab some tea but I'm already having trouble. My young friend and I jog up the long hill over 128 to the Newton-Wellesley Hospital. He gets slower and slower and finally says he'll walk a while and catch up, but I never see him again.

The traffic is very heavy and the thick fumes of unburnt exhaust catch in the dryness of my throat. Turning right on Commonwealth Avenue there is a lot of impatient horn blowing. The hills get harder. I'm lightheaded and my mind blurred and irrational. This is the crisis of a marathon; when your body sugar is gone and the piled-up toxins of exhaustion conspire to destroy your will to go on and random, crazy thoughts run through your mind.

I can't remember feeling as badly as this, even after 20 miles and realize I'm terribly dehydrated. Then as I come up "Heartbreak Hill," I see Susan, like some guardian angel. At the car I gulp a drink and chew a salt pill. Bill says, "You're going great! Only 6 miles more and they're all downhill," which isn't true.

More slugging rain, traffic, and exhaust fumes hang in my nose and lungs. A construction area is a mess of mud and rocks. I pass some runners, now walking, chilled and silent in their skimpy track clothes. My hands are numb as I turn into Beacon Street on the green light. Over a cluster of low buildings the top of the Prudential tower, shadowy in the mist, looks 100 miles away. Susan gives me some gloves and my hands get better, but the blocks crawl by at snail's pace. At 24 miles I pass more walkers in the rain. There's a mass of traffic at Coolidge Corner. I start across against the light as Bill charges out shouting and halts the onrushing tide of traffic. Up over the steep railroad bridge I see a tangle of traffic at Kenmore Square, where it helps with the Boston police if you're lucky enough to have a blonde daughter with a smile like the sun on the Lake of Killarney. The holiday traffic is like Broadway and 42nd Street with Wiltshire Boulevard through the middle, and the late runner hasn't a chance. But Susan has put a spell on the officer, who raises both arms, blasting on his whistle. All traffic halts while I slog through.

Under the overhead ramp from Storrow Drive there's Charlesgate East. I feel like dying, yet elated, because now I know I can make it. A right turn against traffic, and I pass one more hobbling walker. Across Boylston Street up on the Plaza Road and I finish as fast as I can go.

All at once the horrors of the last 5 miles are forgotten and my aching legs are ignored. I'm floating on air and want to grab the first stranger in the street and tell him I've just run the Boston Marathon.

Standing there in the drizzle in front of the vast Prudential building, I turn and gaze up at the muscular statue of a bronze god, who spurts up from his pedestal to preside over the exhausted runners as they cross the finish line. Appropriately named *Quest Eternal,* by Donald DeLue, he measures 26 miles, 385 yards from Hopkinton, but from the start of training he's more like 3,000 miles away.

This story is a joke to any serious marathon runner and a matter of controversy with officials of the Boston Athletic Association, who have eliminated many of us with the 3½-hour limit for their world-famous and charismatic race. But to me or any other jogger who completes a marathon there is a reward that can't be described in words, and even without Boston, I can still run in the other marathons and be greeted at the finish by my children and grandchildren.

In the last few years, races have sprung up all over the country. There are hundreds of 10-mile, 20–30 kilometer, and, as you improve, 20-mile races. Then, for the well-trained runner, there are over 150 marathons alone. There are joggers' and plodders' races, where benign officials don't mind waiting long after the winners until you come in. The sport is growing and maybe some day there will be races in every community for all ages and all comers, and jogging trails from Presque Isle, Maine, to San Diego, California.

In Conclusion

Psychologists and sociologists say that the sickness in our society and its fragmentation into thousands of movements and subcults is caused by the dire need of confused individuals to belong to something to which they can relate and which will provide them with a sense of security and fulfillment. The beauty of the life style we have offered you is that it brings not only this sense of security, but in no other way can you achieve these other enormous benefits that make up the base, the foundation for everything else you do in life. For example:

Action

Here is the way to counteract, with a vigorous, active life, the sedentary influences of technology and at the same time act out in a physical sense the glandular responses to the stresses and tensions of our fast-changing society.

Food

Use delicious, healthful nutrition to replace those empty foods that are destroying us in a physical sense. The American diet of cola drinks, hamburgers, french fries, white bread, thick greasy sauces, and rich desserts is a nutritional disaster that is equivalent to slow murder or suicide, depending on whether you are cooking or eating.

Relationship

Here is a life style that gives immediate identity and after a relatively short time new confidence and self-assurance that will be felt both by others and by its possessor. It has worked for us and it has worked for millions of others who have joined the fitness and health movement. These new arrivals come through many different sources—through the health food culture, through ecology and the environment, through the influence of doctors, coaches, and from simple enthusiasts like ourselves. But whatever the source, to our great delight the movement is growing by leaps and bounds.

    These are people who have learned how to live in balance with our changing environment. They have gained both emotional maturity and a kind of spiritual strength, which enable them to keep their perspective and a sense of well-being in this confusing and turbulent world.

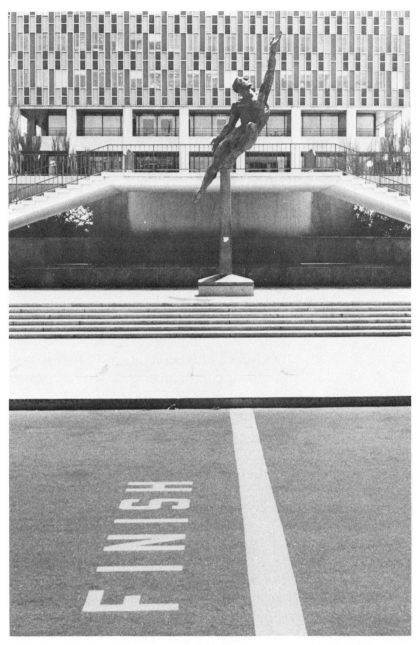

Quest Eternal, by Donald DeLue, presides over finish line of Boston Marathon.

Appendix
Glossary
References
Index

Appendix

AVERAGE AMOUNT OF CALORIES EXPENDED FOR VARIOUS ACTIVITIES

(These are approximate average values for someone weighing 140–150 lbs. They include the energy needed for basal metabolism.)

Activity			Hour	*Calories Per:* Half-hour	Minute
Sleeping (for comparison)			75	38	1.25
RECREATION AND EXERCISE					
Walking on level	2.0	mph	180	90	3.00
	3.0	mph	260	130	4.33
	3.5	mph	300	150	5.00
	4.0	mph	350	175	5.83
	4.5	mph	480	240	8.00
	5.3	mph	620	310	10.33
Walking upstairs	1.0	mph	195	98	3.25
	2.0	mph	640	320	10.67
Walking downstairs	2.0	mph	215	108	3.58
Running on level	5.5	mph	660	330	11.00
	7.2	mph	720	360	12.00
	8.0	mph	825	413	13.75
	10.0	mph	1140	570	19.00
	11.4	mph	1390	695	23.17
Hiking (20-lb. pack)	2.5	mph	300	150	5.00
	3.0	mph	312	156	5.20
	3.5	mph	380	190	6.33
	4.0	mph	450	225	7.50

			Calories Per:		
			Hour	*Half-hour*	*Minute*
Hiking (40-lb.	1.0	mph	210	105	3.50
pack)	2.0	mph	270	135	4.50
	3.0	mph	348	174	5.80
	4.0	mph	540	270	9.00
Swimming					
Crawl stroke	0.7	mph	300	150	5.00
	1.0	mph	420	210	7.00
	1.6	mph	700	350	11.67
	1.9	mph	850	425	14.17
	2.2	mph	1600	800	26.67
Breast	0.7	mph	300	150	5.00
stroke	1.0	mph	410	205	6.83
	1.3	mph	600	300	10.00
Side stroke	1.0	mph	550	275	9.17
	1.6	mph	1200	600	20.00
Back stroke	0.8	mph	300	150	5.00
	1.0	mph	450	225	7.50
	1.2	mph	540	270	9.00
	1.33	mph	660	330	11.00
	1.6	mph	800	400	13.33
Bicycling	5.5	mph	240	120	4.00
	9.0	mph	415	208	6.92
	13.0	mph	660	330	11.00
Skiing					
On level	3.0	mph	540	270	9.00
	5.0	mph	720	360	12.00
Downhill	Various		300–500	150–250	5.0–8.33
Skating	Leisurely		350	175	5.83
	9.0	mph	470	235	7.83
	11.0	mph	640	320	10.67
	13.0	mph	780	390	13.00

Activity			Calories Per:		
			Hour	*Half-hour*	*Minute*
Snowshoeing	2.5	mph	620	310	10.33
Rowing	2.5	mph	300	150	5.00
	3.5	mph	660	330	11.00
	11.0	mph	970	485	16.17
Canoeing	Leisurely		230	115	3.83
	4.0	mph	420	210	7.00
Baseball					
(Except pitcher)			300	150	5.00
Pitcher			400	200	6.67
Volleyball					
Recreational			350	175	5.83
Competitive			600	300	10.00
Basketball			608	304	10.13
Tennis					
Recreational			450	225	7.50
Competitive and singles			600	300	10.00
Golf (no carts)			300	150	5.00
Bowling			270	135	4.50
Squash			600–800	300–400	10.00–13.33
Fencing			630	315	10.50
Horseback riding (trot)			415	208	6.92
Badminton					
Recreational			350	175	5.83
Competitive			600	300	10.00
Mountain climbing			600	300	10.00
Table tennis			360	180	6.00
GENERAL FITNESS EXERCISES					
Basic level			200	100	3.33
Intermediate and advanced levels			400	200	6.67

Activity	*Calories Per:*		
	Hour	*Half-hour*	*Minute*
GENERAL			
Lying down	85	43	1.42
Watching TV in chair	107	54	1.78
Mental work (seated)	110	55	1.83
Sewing, handwork	115	58	1.92
Dressing and undressing	140	70	2.33
Driving a car	150	75	2.50
Office work	155	78	2.58
Light housework	165	83	2.75
Ironing	150	75	2.50
Sweeping, vacuuming	180	90	3.00
Cleaning windows	195	98	3.25
Polishing	210	105	3.50
Laundry work	240	120	4.00
Making beds	270	135	4.50
Mopping	300	150	5.00
Gardening	250	125	4.17
House painting	225	113	3.75
Chopping wood	480	240	8.00
Sawing wood	515	258	8.58
Stacking firewood	370	185	6.17
Carpentry work	230	115	3.83
Shoveling dirt	425	213	7.08
Stone masonry	420	210	7.00
Machinist work (light)	180	90	3.00
Printing work	150	75	2.50

Glossary

adrenaline   The proprietary name for *epinephrine;* a hormone produced by the medulla of the adrenal gland. It increases the heart rate, blood pressure, and cardiac output, having the effect of deferring muscular fatigue. It also exerts an influence on the smooth muscles of internal organs. During stress, it is released in larger quantities, thus permitting exceptional amounts of activity.

aerobic exercise   Exercise sufficiently strenuous to create an increased demand for oxygen and to increase the heartbeat and breathing, and which lasts over 5–10 minutes yet does not produce oxygen debt.

atheromatous   The condition or characteristic of fatty deposits of the inner lining of the arteries.

basal metabolism   The quantity of energy used by the body in a fasting and resting state, when it uses just enough to maintain vital cellular activity, respiration, and circulation.

calisthenics   Arm, leg, and body movements without weights.

calorie   The calorie used in metabolism is the amount of heat required to raise the temperature of 1 kilogram of water 1° centigrade, and as a measure of heat is also a measure of the energy properties of food.

capillaries   Minute blood vessels at the end point of the arterial blood supply that deliver oxygen and nutrients to the tissues and pick up waste products and send them back into the veins.

carcinogen   A substance or agent producing cancerous growth.

carcinogenicity   A state or condition producing or tending to produce cancer.

cardiologist   A medical doctor who specializes in the heart and its action, and in the diagnosis and treatment of its diseases.

cardiovascular   Of, relating to, or involving the heart and blood vessels.

cholesterol   A fatlike substance that occurs as an essential constituent of body cells and fluids of all animals. Although it has been implicated experimentally in arteriosclerosis, it is important and necessary in certain physiological processes and is synthesized in the body, especially by the liver and adrenal cortex.

component   A constituent part of any given whole.

coronary disease   Also coronary artery disease or coronary heart disease: A condition that narrows the coronary arteries and thereby reduces the blood flow to the heart muscle.

dehydration   An abnormal depletion of body fluids resulting from high-stress exercise without adequate fluid replacement. (This is a limited definition, as it can come from other causes that are not relevant to this book.)

electrocardiogram   A tracing made by an electrocardiograph, an instrument for recording the changes of electrical potential occurring during the heartbeat; used especially in diagnosing abnormalities of heart action.

electrolyte A substance that, as an acid, base, or salt, becomes an ionic conductor when dissolved in a suitable solvent (in this case, the body fluids).

endocrines Ductless glands that secrete hormones directly into the bloodstream.

equivalent An equivalent, expressed in grams, is the atomic weight divided by the valence.

exercise Any physical activity.

extracellular fluid The portion of total body fluid that is situated outside the cells, and which is subject to most of the shrinkage in dehydration.

homeostasis The tendency in the bodies of higher animals to keep things the way they are, regardless of constant changes in the external and internal environments.

hypertrophy (muscular) Overgrowth or excessive development of the skeletal muscles.

hypocholesterolemic The characteristic of an activity, a particular diet, or a drug that tends to decrease the cholesterol concentration of the blood. (Limited definition.)

hypotonic Having a lower amount in solution of a given substance or electrolyte than the body fluids to which it is being compared. (Limited definition.)

metabolism The sum of the processes and chemical changes in living cells by which energy is provided for the vital activities and new material is assimilated for repair and wastes are removed.

milliequivalent (abbrev. meq) One-thousandth of an equivalent of a chemical element, radical, or compound.

saline Consisting of, or containing salt (sodium chloride) or other salts of sodium and of calcium, magnesium, or potassium. (Limited definition.)

saturated fat or *fatty acid* The type of dietary fat found principally in animal fats that tends to increase blood cholesterol and is considered to cause dangerous fatty deposits in the walls of the arteries. (Simplified definition limited to the aspect of the subject with which we are concerned in this book.)

somatotype   Soma (body) plus type, physique; a classification of human body-build in terms of the relative development of ectomorphic, endomorphic, and mesomorphic components.

unsaturated fat or *polyunsaturated fat* or *fatty acid*   The type of dietary fat found principally in vegetables, seeds, and their products, in certain fish and, to a lesser extent, in poultry; is now considered to have a reducing effect on blood cholesterol and hence avoid the harmful fatty deposits in the walls of arteries caused by saturated fat. (This is a very simplified, limited definition.)

weight lifting   Movements with heavy and extremely heavy weights (with which this book is not concerned).

weight training   Arm, leg, and body movements with light to medium weights.

Selected References

Introduction

Discussion of resting and standing heart rates: William V. Beshlian, M.D., personal communication on the causes of low resting heart rates.

The efficiency of the slow-beating heart: Lawrence E. Lamb, M.D., *Your Heart and How to Live With It* (New York: Viking Press, 1969), pp. 47, 138–140, 154.

Physiological differences between trained and untrained individuals, including outstanding athletes: Ross A. McFarland, Ph.D., *Human Factors in Air Transportation* . . . (New York: McGraw-Hill, 1953), pp. 272–277.

"The Physical Examination," and "Guidelines in the Management of the Exercising Patient": Kenneth H. Cooper,

M.D., M.P.H., *The New Aerobics* (New York: M. Evans and Co., 1970), pp. 21–23.

Chapter 2

For applicable energy values for calorie surplus chart, see references for Appendix.

Dale Groom, M.D., F.A.C.P., "Cardiovascular Observations on Tarahumara Indian Runners—The Modern Spartans," *American Heart Journal,* Vol. 81, No. 3 (March, 1971), pp. 304–314.

Bodily response to emotions is covered in Walter B. Cannon, M.D., S.D., LL.D., *Bodily Changes in Pain, Hunger, Fear and Rage* (College Park, Md.: McGrath Publishing Co., 1929, reprinted 1970), pp. 49–65, 258–267.

The "fight or flight" response with lack of activity; if unreleased, these unused energies can cause emotional and physical disturbances: Hans Kraus, M.D., *Backache, Stress and Tension* (New York: Simon and Schuster, 1965), pp. 66–72.

The ability of the body to adapt to stress and hardship: Hans Selye, M.D., *The Stress of Life* (New York: McGraw-Hill, 1956), p. 119.

A study of intensely active Swiss mountain populations with a high intake of dairy fats and a low mortality from cardiovascular disease: F. Verzar, and D. Gsell, *Ernahrung und Gesundheitszustand der Bergbevlkerung der Schweiz* (Bern, Switzerland: H. Tschudy and Co., 1962).

A blood cholesterol study of very active Swiss mountain people. Daniella Gsell, M.D. and Jean Mayer, Ph.D., D.Sc., "Low Blood Cholesterol Associated with High-Calorie, High-Saturated Fat Intakes in a Swiss Alpine Population," *The American Journal of Clinical Nutrition,* Vol. 10, No. 6 (June, 1962), pp. 471–479.

The Irish brothers study: F. J. Stare, M.D., "Comparisons of

Siblings in Boston and Ireland," *Journal of the American Dietetic Association,* Vol. 45, No. 3 (September, 1964).

The deterioration of the astronauts due to weightlessness: Earl W. Brannon, USAF-MC; Captain Charles A. Rockwood, Jr., USAF-MC; Major Pauline Potts, USAF-MSC, "The Influence of Specific Exercises in the Prevention of Debilitating Musculoskeletal Disorders; Implication in Physiological Conditioning for Prolonged Weightlessness," *Aerospace Medicine,* Vol. 34 (October, 1963), p. 900.

"Current Research on Sleep and Dreams," U.S. Department of Health, Education, and Welfare, *Public Health Service Publication No. 1389,* 1971, Chapter IV, Sleep Disorders, pp. 28–29.

Rest value gained from just lying there. Warren R. Guild, M.D., Samm Sinclair Baker, and Stuart D. Cowan, *Vigor for Men Over 30* (New York: Macmillan, 1967), p. 154.

For physiological characteristics in acclimatization to high altitude, see: David Bruce Dill, Ph.D., *Life, Heat and Altitude* . . . (Cambridge, Mass.: Harvard University Press, 1938), pp. 150, 157, 162, 167; and Ross A. McFarland, Ph.D., *Human Factors in Air Transportation* . . . (New York: McGraw-Hill, 1953), pp. 235–237.

Chapter 3

Freud's *Drei Abhandlungen zur Sexualtheorie,* first published in 1905, was translated by Brill in 1910 and published as *Three Contributions to the Sexual Theory.*

For explanation of the child's attempts at locomotion, see: Franz Alexander, M.D., *The Fundamentals of Psychoanalysis* (New York: Norton, 1948), pp. 41–43.

For the child and the adult within us, see: Thomas A. Harris, M.D., *I'm OK—You're OK* (New York and Evanston: Harper and Row, 1969), Chapter 2.

The early myth of Eros varies according to different philosophers, poets, or mythologians. This version derived from: H. A. Guerber, revised by Dorothy Margaret Stuart, *The Myths of Greece and Rome* (London: George C. Harrap and Co., 1960), p. 12.

Chapter 5

Food intake must be balanced to energy output: Jean Mayer, Ph.D., D.Sc., *Overweight Causes, Cost, and Control* (Englewood Cliffs, N.J.: Prentice-Hall, 1968), pp. 124–125.

Endurance exercise builds collateral circulation and keeps healthy blood vessels soft and pliable: Thomas K. Cureton, *The Physiological Effects of Exercise Programs on Adults* (Springfield, Ill.: Charles C. Thomas, 1969), pp. 33–41; and John L. Boyer, M.D., American College of Sports Medicine, Address at Masters Track and Field Meet, San Diego, Calif., July 5, 1970.

Exercise keeps bones strong: Per-Olof Åstrand, M.D. and Kaare Rodahl, M.D., *Textbook of Work Physiology* (New York: McGraw-Hill, 1970), pp. 260–262, 418–420.

Exercise helps you to eat in balance with your output: *Ibid.,* pp. 473–475.

Musculature of weight lifters covered in: Charles Palmer, *Exercises for Runners* (Mountain View, Calif.: World Publications, 1973), pp. 50–53.

The tendency to "store" with missed meals is discussed in: E. S. Gordon, M.D., Marshall Goldberg, M.D., and Grace J. Chosy, B.S., "A New Concept in the Treatment of Obesity," *Journal of the American Medical Association,* Vol. 186, No. 1 (October 5, 1963), pp. 158, 161–165.

The difference between sports or recreation and aerobic or cardiopulmonary exercise: Kenneth H. Cooper, M.D., M.P.H., *Aerobics* (New York: M. Evans and Co., 1968), pp. 31–43.

The tremendous importance of "steady state," aerobic, or cardiovascular exercise is well covered in: Ross A. McFarland, Ph.D., *Human Factors in Air Transportation* . . . (New York: McGraw-Hill, 1953), pp. 272–277.

The need for calisthenics and weight training as a supplement to CPE: Charles T. Kuntzleman, Ph.D., ed., *The Physical Fitness Encyclopedia* (Emmaus, Pa.: Rodale Books, 1970), pp. 539–541.

Fred Wilt, *Run Run Run* (Los Altos, Calif.: Track and Field News, 1970), pp. 42, 43, 89, 108, 117, 136, 165.

Chapter 7

The mechanics of lifting heavy weights: Per-Olof Åstrand, M.D. and Kaare Rodahl, M.D., *Textbook of Work Physiology* (New York: McGraw-Hill, 1970), pp. 271–275.

Chapter 8

For the Cooper point system for aerobic exercise see: Kenneth H. Cooper, M.D., M.P.H., *The New Aerobics* (New York: M. Evans and Co., 1970), p. 172.

The use of light exercise using other muscle groups to promote recovery and avoid soreness of muscles: Per-Olof Åstrand, M.D. and Kaare Rodahl, M.D., *Textbook of Work Physiology* (New York: McGraw-Hill, 1970), p. 91.

Chapter 9

The dangers of "cut-out" diets: Jean Mayer, Ph.D., D.Sc., *Overweight Causes, Cost, and Control* (Englewood Cliffs, N.J.: Prentice-Hall, 1968), pp. 4–5.

The comment about *Dr. Atkins Diet Revolution* is from *Today's Health* (April 1974), p. 56.

Low-calorie consumers need to increase physical activity so
they can eat more and get enough nutrients: Per-Olof Ås-
trand, M.D. and Kaare Rodahl, M.D., *Textbook of Work
Physiology* (New York: McGraw-Hill, 1970), pp. 471–473.
The problem with high-calorie deficits: Warren R. Guild, M.D.,
Robert E. Fuisz, M.D., and Samuel Bojar, M.D., *The Science of Health* (Englewood Cliffs, N.J.: Prentice-Hall,
1969), pp. 326–327.
Homeostasis is discussed in: Jean Mayer, Ph.D., D.Sc., *Over-
weight Causes, Cost, and Control* (Englewood Cliffs, N.J.:
Prentice-Hall, 1968), pp. 12–15; 24–25.
The relationship of calorie deficits to weight loss and the dangers
of crash diets: Frederick J. Stare, M.D., *Eating for Good
Health* (Garden City, N.Y.: Doubleday, 1964 and 1968), pp.
179–180.
The need for more small meals per day rather than fewer large
ones: the problem of skipping meals: Jean Mayer, Ph.D.,
D.Sc., *Overweight Causes, Cost, and Control* (Englewood
Cliffs, N.J.: Prentice-Hall, 1968), pp. 159–160 and p. 203,
par. 49.
Eating slowly gives satiety gland time to work: *Ibid.,* pp. 196–
197. Exercise does not necessarily increase food intake:
Ibid., pp. 69, 72.
The Seven Food Groups have been expanded from the traditional four to provide a better distribution of nutrients.
Many families tend to shop for their food in a pattern, so
that they buy repetitiously and eat more than they need of
some nutrients and less than they need of others. One of the
objectives in Chapter 9 is to help them break out of that pattern. For example, a study of the tables in *Composition of
Foods,* Agriculture Handbook No. 8, USDA, 1963 (referred to below as *Composition of Foods*) and the *Heinz
Handbook of Nutrition* (New York: The Blakiston Division, McGraw-Hill, 1965) indicates that better nutrition results from a diet with both fruit and vegetables, rather than

a diet (a) with vegetables only, or (b) with fruit only. The same holds true of meat, fish, and poultry.

References concerning the three important concepts are as follows:

1. Frederick J. Stare, M.D., *Eating for Good Health* (Garden City, N.Y.: Doubleday, 1964 and 1968) p. 180.
Per-Olof Åstrand, M.D. and Kaare Rodahl, M.D., *Textbook of Work Physiology* (New York: McGraw-Hill, 1970) p. 473.

2. Roger J. Williams, Ph.D., D.Sc., *Nutrition Against Disease, Environmental Prevention* (New York: Pitman Publishing Corp., 1971), p. 247, ref. 34; and p. 249, ref. 43.

3. Jean Mayer, Ph.D., D.Sc., *Overweight Causes, Cost, and Control* (Englewood Cliffs, N.J.: Prentice-Hall, 1968), pp. 136, 143, and D. M. Hegsted, Ph.D., Department of Nutrition, Harvard School of Public Health, "Protein needs and possible modifications of the American diet," Journal of The American Dietetic Association, Vol. 68, April 1976, p. 320, discusses the need to reduce consumption of meat and fat, particularly saturated fat and cholesterol with greater consumption of vegetables, fruits and cereals.

For ways to handle low fat cooking, see: Evelyn S. Stead, and Gloria K. Warren, *Low Fat Cookery* (New York: McGraw-Hill, 1956, 1959).

For effects of heat treatment of edible oils, see: Roger J. Williams, Ph.D., D.Sc., *Nutrition Against Disease, Environmental Prevention* (New York: Pitman Publishing Corp., 1971), pp. 269–270.

For comprehensive discussion of protein, see: Benjamin T. Burton, *The Heinz Handbook of Nutrition,* Second Edition (New York: The Blakiston Division, McGraw-Hill, 1965), pp. 45–51.

For composition of "Incaparina," see *Ibid.,* pp. 238–239.

Net Protein Utilization is explained in: Frances Moore Lappé,

Diet for a Small Planet (New York: Ballantine Books, 1971, revised 1975), pp. 61–85.

The method of balancing vegetable protein to obtain optimum biologic value is explained in: *Ibid.,* Part III, pp. 89–134.

Recommended Dietary Allowances from *Journal of the American Dietetic Association,* Vol. 64, No. 2, February, 1974.

For nutritional values of wheat bran, see: *Composition of Foods,* item no. 2446, "Wheat bran," p. 66; see also item 1880, "Rice bran," p. 52.

Dr. Burkitt's paper was reported in *Medical Tribune,* Vol. 12, No. 5 (February 3, 1971), "A Refined Carbohydrate Diet is Linked with Colon Cancer." *Ibid.,* editorial February 24, 1971.

Removal of fiber in foods linked to diseases of Western societies: Denis P. Burkitt, M.D., "The Importance of Fibre in Food." *Bulletin No. 7,* British Nutrition Foundation, May, 1972, pp. 29–35.

The nutritional deficiency of commercial white bread. Roger J. Williams, Ph.D., D.Sc., *Nutrition Against Disease, Environmental Prevention* (New York: Pitman Publishing Corp., 1971), pp. 200–201 and p. 298, references 2 and 3.

Improvement of Bread: *Ibid.,* pp. 198–205.

Nutritional sense and nonsense about food fads: *Ibid.,* Chapter 13.

The loss of nutrition in processing. Carl C. Pfeiffer, Ph.D., M.D., *Mental and Elemental Nutrients* (New Canaan, Conn.: Keats Publishing, 1975), pp. 24–27, 174.

For discussion of sugar content of commercial breakfast cereals, see *Ibid.,* p. 28.

Inaccuracy of advertising claims of some packaged dry cereals reported by Robert B. Choate, Testimony before Subcommittee on the Consumer Committee on Commerce, United States Senate, July 23, 1970.

Increase in cadmium-zinc ratio from processing, a factor in high blood pressure and kidney disorders, is from: Henry A.

Schroeder, M.D., Alexis P. Nason, B.A., Isabel H. Tipton, Ph.D., and Joseph J. Balassa, Ph.D., *Essential Trace Metals in Man: Zinc. Relation to Environmental Cadmium* (Great Britain: Pergamon Press, J. Chron. Dis., Vol. 20, 1967), pp. 179–210, and Henry A. Schroeder, "Cadmium, Chromium and Cardiovascular Disease," The George E. Brown Memorial Lecture, October 22, 1966; Circulation in Press.

For zinc content of wheat bran and other foods, see: Carl C. Pfeiffer, Ph.D., M.D., *Mental and Elemental Nutrients* (New Canaan, Conn., Keats Publishing, 1975), Table 16.3, pp. 241–242.

Coconut oil is 92 percent saturated fat, butterfat is 58 percent. Ancel and Margaret Keys, *Eat Well and Stay Well* (Garden City, N.Y.: Doubleday, 1963), pp. 352–353.

Cholesterol in human milk and in cow's milk. Raymond Reiser, Ph.D., Texas A&M University, *Focus,* publication of National Dairy Council, Vol. X, No. 3 (February 3, 1969).

Milk fat and processed milk. Roger J. Williams, Ph.D., D.Sc., *Nutrition Against Disease, Environmental Prevention* (New York: Pitman Publishing Corp., 1971), pp. 268–269.

Protein content of various cuts of beef. *Composition of Foods,* pp. 11–15.

Implication of chemicals used in processing smoked meats. Melvin Greenblatt, M.D., Sidney Mirvish, Ph.D., and Bing T. So, M.D., The Eppley Institute for Research in Cancer, University of Nebraska College of Medicine, "Nitrosamine Studies: Induction of Lung Adenomas by Concurrent Administration of Sodium Nitrite and Secondary Amines in Swiss Mice," *Journal of National Cancer Institute,* Vol. 46, pp. 1029–1034 (1971).

For report on mercury and other contaminants in fish, see: Frances Moore Lappé, *Diet for a Small Planet* (New York: Ballantine Books, 1971), pp. 36–37, 96, 130, 137.

Cholesterol content of eggs: *Composition of Foods,* p. 146.

Nutritional composition of eggs: *Ibid.,* p. 30.

Rate of cholesterol synthesis in the body: Roger J. Williams, Ph.D., D.Sc., *Nutrition Against Disease, Environmental Prevention* (New York: Pitman Publishing Corp., 1971), p. 239, ref. 11.

Crystalline cholesterol: Mark D. Altschule, M.D., "On the Much-Maligned Egg," from *Executive Health,* Vol. X, No. 8 (1974).

Additional vitamins of certain types advisable in high-output exercise programs: Thomas K. Cureton, Ph.D., F.A.C.S.M., "Diet Makes a Difference," *Fitness for Living,* May–June, 1969, pp. 57–60.

Excess of Vitamin A and Vitamin D can cause toxicity: Abraham White, Philip Handler, and Emil L. Smith, *Principles of Biochemistry* (New York: McGraw-Hill, [3rd Edition], 1968), p. 894.

Foods fried in saturated fat can be harmful: Jean Mayer, Ph.D., D.Sc., "How to Murder Your Husband," *Family Health,* May, 1970.

Alcohol interferes with the delivery of oxygen to the cells and impairs performance: Kenneth H. Cooper, M.D., M.P.H., *Aerobics* (New York: M. Evans and Co., 1968), p. 220.

The sludging effect of alcohol in the capillaries: Herbert A. Moskow, Raymond C. Pennington, and Melvin H. Knisely, "Alcohol, Sludge and Hypoxic Areas of Nervous System, Liver and Heart," *Microvascular Research,* 1 (March 18, 1968), pp. 174–185.

Sugar furnishes empty calories. Ancel and Margaret Keys, *Eat Well and Stay Well* (Garden City, N.Y.: Doubleday [2nd ed.], 1963), pp. 161–162.

Chapter 10

The various body types and the tendency of mesomorphs to cardiovascular disease: William H. Sheldon, Ph.D., M.D.,

Atlas of Men (Darien, Conn.: Hafner Publishing Co., 1954 [reprinted 1970]), pp. 62, 115, 176, 185; and the qualities of the ectomorph: *Ibid.*, pp. 36, 38, 47, 51.

The significance of added bone from the standpoint of structural strength: Per-Olof Åstrand, M.D. and Kaare Rodahl, M.D., *Textbook of Work Physiology* (New York: McGraw-Hill, 1970), pp. 260–263; 418–420.

The breakdown of component weights of the sedentary man and the active man is from: Josef Brozek et al., "Body Composition, Part I," *Annals of New York Academy of Science,* Vol. 110 (September 26, 1963), p. 195.

Skinfold tests as a measure of obesity: Jean Mayer, Ph.D., D.Sc., *Overweight Causes, Cost, and Control* (Englewood Cliffs, N.J.: Prentice-Hall, 1968), pp. 29–34.

Use of Lange constant-pressure caliper in skinfold tests: Carl C. Seltzer, Howard W. Stoudt, and Benjamin Bell, "Reliability of Relative Body Weight as a Criterion of Obesity," *American Journal of Epidemiology,* Vol. 92, No. 6 (1970), pp. 340–349.

The average waist measurements of both male and female samples are from: Howard W. Stoudt, Ph.D., Albert Damon, Ph.D., and Ross A. McFarland, Ph.D., Harvard University, and Jean Roberts, Division of Health Examination Statistics, "Skinfolds, Body Girths, Biacromial Diameter, and Selected Anthropometric Indices of Adults, United States, 1960–1962," *Public Health Service Publication No. 1000—Series 11—No. 35,* U.S. Department of Health, Education and Welfare, pp. 21–22.

Chapter 11

"Physiological Effects in Hot Climates," David Bruce Dill, Ph.D., *Life, Heat and Altitude* . . . (Cambridge, Mass.: Harvard University Press, 1938), Chapters I, II, and III.

Recommendations for fluid and electrolyte replacement are

in: Richard L. Westerman, M.D., "Fluid and Electrolyte Replacement in Sweating Athletes," and "Percutaneous vs. Perpulmonic Loss of Fluid and Electrolytes During Exercise," *Journal of American Medical Association*, Vol. 212, No. 10 (June 8, 1970), pp. 1713–1714; *Ibid.*, personal communications.

Definitions and discussion of heat illness are adapted from: *Webster's Third New International Dictionary, Unabridged* (Merriam-Webster) (Springfield, Mass.: G. & C. Merriam Company, Publishers, 1966), and from: *Encyclopedia of Sports Sciences and Medicine*, Leonard A. Larson, Ph.D., executive editor (New York: Macmillan, 1971), p. 1526.

Discussion of acclimatization, and fluid and electrolyte procedures are from: Gerard Balakian, M.D., F.C.P., "Action Aid for Athletes," *The Journal of the Medical Society of New Jersey*, Vol. 67, No. 9 (September 1970), pp. 517–522; and *Ibid.*, "What are the 'Ades' all About?" *Medical Times*, Vol. 99, No. 9 (September 1971), page 202; and Richard L. Westerman, M.D., personal communications.

There should be no restrictions on taking fluid at any time: C. H. Wyndham, and M. B. Strydom, "The Danger of an Inadequate Water Intake During Marathon Running," *South African Medical Journal*, Vol. 43 (July–December, 1969 and Supplements), pp. 893–896.

Salt tablets must be taken with adequate water. Richard L. Westerman, M.D., "Fluid and Electrolyte Replacement in Sweating Athletes," *Journal of American Medical Association*, Vol. 212, No. 10 (June 8, 1970), pp. 1713–1714.

Water alone can cause cramps: Gerard Balakian, M.D., "What are the 'Ades' all About?" *Medical Times*, Vol. 99, No. 9 (September 1971), p. 202.

Discussion of rates of gastric emptying: John S. Fordtran and Bengt Saltin, "Gastric Emptying and Intestinal Absorption During Prolonged Severe Exercise," *Journal of Applied Physiology*, Vol. 23, No. 3 (September 1967), pp. 331–335.

Dr. Costill's comments on water and salt loss, and decreased muscle sugar are in: David L. Costill, Ph.D., *What Research Tells the Coach about Distance Running* (Washington, D.C.: American Association of Health, Physical Education and Recreation, 1968), pp. 34–35.

Control of body temperatures by transfer of heat through the skin: *Ibid.,* pp. 41–42.

Reduction in blood volume caused by dehydration: *Ibid.,* p. 43.

Rectal temperatures of marathon runners in the heat: *Ibid.,* p. 42.

Composition of sea salt is from: *The New International Encyclopedia* (New York: Dodd, Mead and Co., 1930), Vol. 17, pp. 352–353.

The need for magnesium is discussed by Kenneth H. Cooper, M.D., M.P.H., *Runner's World* (November 1971), p. 37 and in: "Low Calorie Diet May Result in Magnesium Lag in Athlete," *Medical Tribune,* August 11, 1971.

Electrolyte values are from: *Composition of Foods.*

Dr. Hursch's comments are from: Laurence M. Hursch, M.D., "Nutrition in the Athlete," Summer Conference of the National Dairy Council, Chicago, June 10, 1968.

Dr. Bass's position was stated in a personal communication. Composition of Body Fluids: Abraham White, Philip Handler, and Emil L. Smith, *Principles of Biochemistry* (New York: McGraw-Hill [3rd Edition], 1968), pp. 778–780.

Chapter 12

Emotional stress can cause physical illness: Walter C. Alvarez, M.D., Mayo Clinic, is quoted in "The Human Situation, About Peptic Ulcers . . . ," *Executive Health,* Vol. VI, No. 12 (1970), p. 4.

Mental health and physical fitness; exercise is of help with psychic tensions: V. B. O. Hammett, M.D., "Psychological Changes with Physical Fitness Training," *Canadian Medi-*

cal Association Journal, Vol. 96, March 25, 1967, pp.
764–766.

"Maintenance of Physical and Psychological Fitness in Air
Crews," Ross A. McFarland, Ph.D., *Human Factors in
Air Transportation* . . . (New York: McGraw-Hill, 1953),
pp. 269–270, 272–277.

Relationship between psychic tension and physical pain and
distress: Walter B. Cannon, M.D., S.D., LL.D., *Bodily
Changes in Pain, Hunger, Fear and Rage* (College Park,
Md.: McGrath Publishing Co., 1929, reprinted 1970), pp.
253–257.

Physical fitness and mental health: Kenneth H. Cooper, M.D.,
M.P.H., *Aerobics* (New York: M. Evans and Co., 1968),
pp. 206–207.

For discussion of somatic compliance, see: Sigmund Freud,
M.D., the Standard Edition of the *Complete Psychological
Works of Sigmund Freud,* trans. and ed. by James Strachey
in collaboration with Anna Freud, Volume VII (London:
Hogarth Press and the Institute of Psycho-Analysis, 1953),
pp. 40–41.

Although not a medical or scientific book, Cameron Hawley's,
The Hurricane Years (Little, Brown and Co., 1968), gives a
most penetrating analysis of the "A" behavior pattern,
which is currently receiving much attention as one of the
causative factors in heart attacks. These authors have been
unable to locate any study or studies that definitively pin
down "Dr. Kharr's" theory that there is an inverse relationship between the production of heparin and the production
of adrenaline; or what it is that stimulates the production of
heparin in the absence of the production of adrenaline.
Therefore, we can only offer this concept as an interesting
and exciting hypothesis, worthy of further research.

Sustained physical activity increases ability to withstand stress
and promotes mental and emotional well-being: Charles T.
Kuntzleman, Ph.D., ed., *The Physical Fitness Encyclo-*

pedia (Emmaus, Pa.: Rodale Books, 1970), pp. 291–292, 390–391.

Appendix

The energy costs of the various activities were selected from tables in the following:

Per-Olof Åstrand, M.D. and Kaare Rodahl, M.D., *Textbook of Work Physiology* (New York: McGraw-Hill, 1970), pp. 438–441.

Benjamin T. Burton, Ph.D., *The Heinz Handbook of Nutrition* (New York: The Blakiston Division, McGraw-Hill, 1959, 1965), p. 27.

Ancel and Margaret Keys, *Eat Well and Stay Well* (Garden City, N.Y.: Doubleday, 1959, 1963), pp. 83–84.

Charles T. Kuntzleman, Ph.D., ed., *The Physical Fitness Encyclopedia* (Emmaus, Pa.: Rodale Books, 1970), pp. 135–137.

Jean Mayer, Ph.D., D.Sc., *Overweight Causes, Cost, and Control* (Englewood Cliffs, N.J.: Prentice-Hall, 1968), pp. 125, 170–171.

John Patrick O'Shea, *Scientific Principles and Methods of Strength Fitness* (Reading, Mass.: Addison-Wesley Publishing Company, 1969), p. 115.

Abraham White, Philip Handler, and Emil L. Smith, *Principles of Biochemistry* (New York: McGraw-Hill [3rd Edition], 1968), pp. 299–300.

A complete list of references is available from the authors upon request.

Index

Boldface numbers refer to illustrations. References to tabular material are followed by the letter t.

172t; composition of, 141, 143,
154–155t, 156, 157t; cooking,
175–176; dairy products, 159t,
160; diet, balanced, 172–175;
fish, 168–169, 169t; fruits, 161–
162, 161–162t; meats, 166–168,
167t; poultry and eggs, 170–
171, 171t; protein, 145–148,
148t; vegetables, 163–166,
163–165t; whole grains and
cereals, 149–159, 149t, 154–
155t, 156–157t
Freud, Dr. Sigmund, 22
Fruits, 161–162, 161–162t

GFE, *see* General Fitness Exer-
cises
General Fitness Exercises,
38–41, 42–77, calories ex-
pended, 235–238t; Alternate
Knee Raise, 46–47, **46–47;** Arms
Flinging, 42–43, **42–43;** Back
Exercises, 54–59, **54–59;**
Double Knee Raise, 48–49,
48–49; Easy Pull-Ups, 69–71,
69–71; Figure 8, 60–63, **60–63;**
Half Knee Bends, 66–68, **66–68;**
Hands Overhead, Swinging to
the Floor, 50–53, **50–53;** Knee
Extension and Flexion, 44–45,
44–45; Push-Ups, 72–74, **72–74;**
Schedule for exercising,
76–77t; Sit-Ups, 64–65, **64–65;**
Time Frame for exercising, 39,
77t, 118t; weight training, *see*
Weight Training
Gookin, Bill, 208
Gordon, Dr. E. S., 142
Graham, Sylvester, 151
Grains, *see* Whole grains
Greek mythology, 21–22, 26
Gsell, Daniella, 15
Guild, Dr. Warren R., 29–30,
225

Harris, Dr. Thomas, 24–25
Hawley, Cameron, 217–218
Hawthorne, Nathaniel, 211
Health, test to determine, xviii
Heart disease survey, 15
Heat illness, 191–195, 197
Hellerstein, Dr. Herman K., 10
Heparin, 218, 256
Hepatitis, 168
Hidgon, Hal, 223
Hill, Ron, 225, 226
Homeostasis, 139–140; and body
weight, 189
Huckleberry Finn (Twain), 214
Hurricane Years, The (Hawley),
217–218
Hursch, Dr. Lawrence M.,
204–205
Hypertonic, 201
Hypertrophy, muscular, 35
Hypocholesterolemic, 158

I'm OK, You're OK (Harris),
24–25
Inactivity and technology, 7–8,
13–14, 15–16; and calorie
surplus, 8–10, 9–10t
"Incaparina," 147
Indians, Tarahumara, 12
"Inferno" (Dante), 217

Jogging, 119–125
Jung, Carl, 24

Kennedy, John F., 212
Ketones, 137
Knee Exercises, Alternate Knee
Raise, 46–47, **46–47;** Double
Knee Raise, 48–49, **48–49;** Half-
Knee Bends, 66–68, **66–68,**
with barbell, 89–91, **89–90;**
Knee Extension and Flexion,
44–45, **44–45**